THE BARBARA KRAUS CHOLESTEROL COUNTER

Other books by Barbara Kraus

The Dictionary of Sodium, Fats, and Cholesterol

Calories and Carbohydrates

The Barbara Kraus Calorie Guide to
Brand Names and Basic Foods

The Barbara Kraus Carbohydrate Guide to
Brand Names and Basic Foods

The Barbara Kraus Dictionary of Protein

The Barbara Kraus Guide to Fiber in Foods

THE
BARBARA KRAUS
CHOLESTEROL COUNTER

BY BARBARA KRAUS

A Perigee Book

Perigee Books
are published by
The Putnam Publishing Group
200 Madison Avenue
New York, NY 10016

Library of Congress Cataloging in Publication Data

Kraus, Barbara.
    The Barbara Kraus Cholesterol counter.

    "A Perigee book."
    1. Food—Cholesterol content—Tables. I. Title.
II. Title: Cholesterol counter.
TX553.C43K73   1985   641.1   84-24841
ISBN 0-399-51134-2

Printed in the United States of America
19 18 17 16 15 14 13 12

For heart patients throughout the world

ABBREVIATIONS AND SYMBOLS

* = prepared as package directs[1]   oz. = ounce
< = less than   pkg. = package
& = and   pt. = pint
" = inch   qt. = quart
canned = bottles or jars as well as cans   sq. = square
dia. = diameter   T. = tablespoon
fl. = fluid   Tr. = trace
liq. = liquid   tsp. = teaspoon
lb. = pound   wt. = weight
med. = medium

All foods not identified by company or trademark brand name have data based on material obtained from the United States Department of Agriculture or Health, Education and Welfare/Food and Agriculture Organization.

EQUIVALENTS

By Weight	By Volume
1 pound = 16 ounces	1 quart = 4 cups
1 ounce = 28.35 grams	1 cup = 8 fluid ounces
3.52 ounces = 100 grams	1 cup = ½ pint
	1 cup = 16 tablespoons
	2 tablespoons = 1 fluid ounce
	1 tablespoon = 3 teaspoons
	1 pound butter = 4 sticks or 2 cups

[1]If the package directions call for whole or skim milk, the data given here are for whole milk unless otherwise stated.

INTRODUCTION

This dictionary lists the total cholesterol content of thousands of food items. Cholesterol has been receiving increasing attention by nutritionists and the medical profession because of its possible relationship to atherosclerosis (coronary heart disease). Of course, diet is not the only factor to be considered in heart disease. Other considerations are heredity, obesity, high blood pressure, blood cholesterol, blood lipids, cigarette smoking, lack of exercise, stress, and certain ailments such as diabetes.

Patients with coronary disease and high blood pressure are often placed on diets in which one or more essential nutrients are controlled. Since physicians now believe that the conditions leading to early heart attacks are the result of a lifetime of habits that predispose individuals to such attacks, they recommend that certain changes in dietary patterns be made also in early childhood.

Cholesterol is one of the complex compounds known as sterols. It is an essential nutrient in normal metabolic processes and is synthesized in the body. It is also present in many foods of animal origin that we consume. Plant foods do not contain cholesterol in any significant amounts. Foods such as chocolate, cocoa, olive oil, coconut butter, and peanut butter are devoid of it since they are plant products.

Animal products are generally high in cholesterol. Organ and glandular meats such as brains, kidney, liver, sweetbreads, and heart are especially high in cholesterol. Egg yolk contains high concentrations of cholesterol, but it is absent in the white.

Cholesterol occurs in both the lean portion and the fatty portions of meat; the removal of fatty tissue if replaced by an equal amount of lean does not reduce the cholesterol intake. This must be taken into account in planning low-cholesterol diets.

Always keep in mind that in making any drastic changes in dietary habits the advice and guidance of a competent physician should be sought. It is essential for good health that the diet contain all the nutrients required by the individual and in adequate amounts. Reductions or increases in one or more of the essential nutrients may bring about adverse effects.

The tables given here are intended to provide basic information to help plan a varied and attractive diet within broad guidelines that are nutritionally adequate when one or more of the essential nutrients must be controlled. This is a comprehensive guide and not an exact quantitative analysis. Quantities may vary slightly from values on labels.

ARRANGEMENT OF THIS BOOK

Foods are listed alphabetically by brand name or by the name of the food. The singular form is used for the entries, that is, blackberry instead of blackberries. Most items are listed individually although a few are grouped. For example, all candies are listed together so that if you are looking for Baby Ruth, you look first under Candy, then under *B* in alphabetical order. But, if you are looking for a breakfast food such as Oatmeal, you will find it under *O* in the main alphabet. Many cross references are included to assist you in finding items known by different names.

Under the main headings, it was often not possible or even desirable to follow an alphabetical arrangement. For basic foods, such as apricots, the first entries are for the fresh product weighed with seeds as it is purchased in the store, then the fruit in small portions as they may be eaten or measured. These entries are followed by the processed products, canned (although it may actually be a bottle or a jar), dehydrated, dried, and frozen items. This basic plan, with adaptations where necessary, was followed for fruits, vegetables, and meats.

In almost all entries, where data were available, the U.S. Department of Agriculture figures are shown first. The department values represent averages from several manufacturers and are shown for comparison with the values from individual companies or for use where particular brands are not available.

Portions Used

The portion column is a most important one to read and note. Common household measures are used wherever possible. For some items, the amounts given are those commonly purchased in the store, such as one pound of meat, or a 15-ounce package of cake mix. These quantities can be divided into the number of servings used in the home and the nutritive values in each portion can then be readily determined. Any ingredients added in preparing such products must also be taken into account.

The smaller portions given are for foods as served or measured in moderate amounts, such as one-half cup of reconstituted juice, or four ounces of meat. Be sure to adjust the amount of the nutrients to the actual portions you use. For example, if you serve one cup of juice instead of one-half cup, multiply the amount of the nutrients shown for the smaller amount by two.

The size of portions you use is extremely important in controlling the intake of any nutrient. The amount of a nutrient is directly related to the weight of the food served. The weight of a volumetric measure, such as a cup or a pint, may vary considerably depending on many factors; four ounces by weight may be very different from one-half cup or four fluid ounces. Ounces in the tables are always ounces by weight unless specified as fluid ounces, fractions of a cup, or other volumetric measure. Foods that are fluffy in texture such as flaked coconut and bean sprouts vary greatly in weight per cup, depending on how tightly they are packed. Such foods as canned green beans also vary when measured with and without liquid; for instance, canned beans with liquid weigh 4.2 ounces for one-half cup, but drained beans weigh 2.5 ounces for the same half cup. Check the weights of your serving portions regularly. Bear in mind that you can reduce or increase the intake of any nutrient by changing the serving size.

It was impossible to convert all the portions to a uniform basis. Some sources were able to report data only in terms of weights with no information on cup or other volumetric measures. We have shown small portions in quantities that one might reasonably expect to be served or measured in the home or institution.

You will find in the portion column the phrases "weighed with bone," and "weighed with skin and seeds." These descriptions apply to the products as you purchase them in the markets, but the nutritive values as shown are for the amount of edible food after you discard the bone, skin, seed, or other inedible part. The weight given in the "measure" or "quantity" column is to the nearest gram or fraction of an ounce.

Data on the composition of foods are constantly changing for many reasons. Better sampling and analytical methods, improvements in marketing procedures, and changes in formulas of mixed products may alter values for all of the nutrients. Weights of packaged foods are frequently changed. It is essential to read label information in order to be knowledgeable about these matters and to make intelligent use of food tables.

A NOTE ON CHOLESTEROL

by James M. Rippe, M.D.
Attending Cardiologist
and
Medical Director, Center for Health,
Fitness and Human Performance
University of Massachusetts Medical School

"What should I do about cholesterol?"

I must get this question a dozen times a week. It is an important question and reflects a growing concern on the part of Americans about diet, exercise and other lifestyle habits. This is a healthy trend and one that members of the medical profession should strongly encourage.

Perhaps no other element of the American diet has engendered such intense concern and controversy as cholesterol. Is cholesterol a friend or a foe? Should all Americans be watching cholesterol, or just a select few? Can you really lower your cholesterol by changing your diet?

While debate rages on in some areas, the evidence in others is overwhelming. I believe we are now in a position to make some unequivocal statements and set some issues to rest.

Elevated blood cholesterol is an established risk factor for coronary heart disease (CHD).

[13]

The average American eats far too much cholesterol and saturated fat (probably *double* the desirable amount).

In individuals with high cholesterol, reduction clearly reduces the likelihood of heart attack.

What is cholesterol? Cholesterol is a naturally occurring waxy substance that performs a number of biological functions. It is needed to make certain hormones and vitamins and also plays a role in cell structure. Some quantity of cholesterol is therefore essential to life. It is only when cholesterol levels become too high that they become a problem. When cholesterol in the blood becomes too high it may be deposited in the walls of the arteries and lead to their narrowing. When it is deposited in the arteries that supply the heart (the coronary arteries) coronary heart disease results.

Cholesterol is both manufactured by the body and obtained from foods. While certain diseases may lead to elevations in blood cholesterol, the vast majority of Americans have elevated cholesterol from increased dietary intake. Cholesterol is one of a class of substances called lipids (triglycerides are another) that result from dietary intake of fats. Fats may be "saturated," "polyunsaturated" or "monosaturated." In general, animal fats are saturated and elevate blood cholesterol while plant fats are unsaturated and cause less elevation or may even lower blood cholesterol.

Cardiologists have been concerned about cholesterol for many years. The link between cholesterol and coronary heart disease has been the subject of continued discussion within the American Heart Association for over two decades. Initial concern emerged from epidemiologic studies that linked elevated blood cholesterol to increased likelihood of developing coronary heart disease. In countries such as Japan where the intake of animal fat (a major source of cholesterol) is significantly lower than in the United States, the CHD is also significantly lower. Interestingly, when Japanese males move to the United States and their dietary intake of fat increases, so do their cholesterol levels and their incidence of coronary heart disease.

Perhaps the most famous study in the United States linking elevated cholesterol to heart disease is the Framingham study. In this study, more than 5,000 men and women in the town of Framingham, Massachusetts, have been followed for over 25 years. Once again, in this study elevated cholesterol is linked to increased incidence of coronary heart disease. Cigarette smoking and hypertension were also established as independent risk factors. Other risk factors include obesity, diabetes, a sedentary lifestyle and stress.

Further evidence linking elevated cholesterol to coronary heart disease has come from animal studies. Until recently, however, one piece of the puzzle has been missing—the piece that proved conclusively that if you actually lowered cholesterol, the chance of heart attack also decreased. Now this final piece has been supplied.

In the recently completed Lipid Research Clinic trial sponsored by the National Heart, Lung and Blood Institute, more than 3,800 men with high cholesterol were followed from 7 to 10 years. The group that took medication to lower cholesterol had 19 percent fewer heart attacks than the other group. Now there is no longer any doubt that individuals with elevated blood cholesterol need to be treated—and treated aggressively. First dietary reduction of cholesterol should be attempted. If significant reductions are not achieved, then a cholesterol-lowering drug should be added.

What does this mean for the average American? Does everyone need to watch cholesterol intake?

There is considerable debate on this subject, but the American Heart Association has recently issued guidelines that seem both reasonable and sane. The AHA recommends that the general public consume a diet with no more than 30 percent of total calories as fat, 55 percent as carbohydrate and 15 percent as protein. The fat should be divided into approximately even portions of saturated, monosaturated and polyunsaturated fatty acids. Cholesterol intake should be limited to less than 300 milligrams per day.

How do Americans stack up against these guidelines? The good news is that more people than ever before are paying attention to what they eat and trying to lower cholesterol intake. Since 1970, the percentage of cholesterol in our diets has steadily declined. The bad news is that it's still far too high. The average American consumes 500 to 600 milligrams of cholesterol a day— almost twice the amount recommended by the AHA! Over 50 percent of middle-aged Americans have cholesterol levels above 200 milligrams per day—above the ideal of 130 to 190 milligrams per day established by the AHA and in the range where the risk of coronary heart disease rapidly increases.

How do you find out what your own cholesterol level is? The simplest way is to have your physician check a blood sample. The AHA recommends that physicians check all individuals for risk factors, and a cholesterol level should certainly be part of this assessment. Don't be lulled into overconfidence by one normal cholesterol reading. Cholesterol readings can vary from test to test and are well known to increase with age. Your level should be checked periodically, at least once every five years after the age of 40.

Even though men have a higher incidence of coronary heart disease, elevated cholesterol is also a risk factor in women, and it is just as important for women to have cholesterol checked as it is for men. What about children? No one knows for sure, but there is increasing evidence that the damage from CHD can begin even in adolescence. Furthermore, childhood is the best time to establish healthy eating habits that will last a lifetime. What about obesity? Weight loss is an important component in lowering cholesterol and attention should be paid to both the number and type of calories ingested.

Will limiting cholesterol in the diet lead to reductions in blood cholesterol? In a word—yes. The average American can expect to achieve a 10 to 15 percent reduction in blood cholesterol by following the AHA guidelines.

All of this brings us to this important book, *The Barbara Kraus Cholesterol Counter*. In order to reduce your dietary intake of cholesterol you must know which foods contain high amounts.

Most Americans are aware that eggs and dairy products are high in cholesterol. Fewer know that red meat constitutes the largest source of cholesterol in the American diet. Fewer still know that organ meats such as liver, brain and kidneys are loaded with cholesterol. High levels of cholesterol can even appear in surprising places. Watch out for that cake mix that calls for an egg or that sauce that's loaded with cream. Processed foods and "fast" foods are also often high in cholesterol.

This handy guide should provide considerable help to every cook and consumer concerned about lowering cholesterol. It comes at a time when increasing attention has been focused on the importance of limiting cholesterol intake. It is a welcome addition.

A

Food and Description	Measure or Quantity	Cholesterol (milligrams)
AC'CENT	¼ tsp.	0
ACEROLA, fresh fruit	Any quantity	0
ALMOND	Any quantity	0
ALMOND EXTRACT	Any quantity	0
AMARANTH	Any quantity	0
ANISE EXTRACT, Virginia Dare, 76% alcohol	1 tsp.	0
APPLE, fresh, canned, dried, or frozen	Any quantity	0
APPLE BUTTER	1 T.	0
APPLE CIDER	Any quantity	0
APPLE JACKS, cereal, Kellogg's	1 cup (1 oz.)	0
APPLE JELLY	Any quantity	0
APPLE JUICE	Any quantity	0
APPLE SAUCE	Any quantity	0
APRICOT, fresh or canned	Any quantity	0

Food and Description	Measure or Quantity	Cholesterol (milligrams)
APRICOT-PINEAPPLE NECTAR	Any quantity	0
APRICOT & PINEAPPLE PRESERVE OR JAM	Any quantity	0
ARBY'S		
Bac'n Cheddar Deluxe	1 sandwich	80
Beef & Cheddar Sandwich	1 sandwich	70
Chicken breast sandwich	7¼-oz. sandwich	56
French Dip	5½-oz. sandwich	55
Ham 'N Cheese	1 sandwich	70
Roast Beef		
Regular	5 oz. sandwich	45
Deluxe	8¼-oz. sandwich	59
Junior	3 oz. sandwich	35
Super	9¼ oz. sandwich	85
Sauce, Horsey	1 oz.	15
Shake		
Chocolate	14-oz. serving	30
Jamocha	14-oz. serving	30
Vanilla	14-oz. serving	35
ARTICHOKE, fresh, canned, or frozen	Any quantity	0
ASPARAGUS, fresh, canned, or frozen	Any quantity	0
AVOCADO, all varieties	Any quantity	0
*AWAKE, Birds Eye	6 fl. (6.5 oz.)	0
AYDS		
Butterscotch, chocolate, or chocolate mint	1 piece (.2 oz.)	Tr.
Vanilla	1 piece (.2 oz.)	1

B

Food and Description	Measure or Quantity	Cholesterol (milligrams)
BACON, broiled, Oscar Mayer		
Regular slice	6-gram slice	5
Thick slice	1 slice (11 grams)	9
Wafer thin	1 slice (4 grams)	3
BACON BITS, Oscar Mayer, real	1 tsp. (2 grams)	2
BACON, CANADIAN, unheated, Oscar Mayer, 93% fat free		
Thin	.7-oz. slice	9
Medium	.8-oz. slice	9
Thick	1-oz. slice	10
BACON, SIMULATED, cooked, Oscar Mayer, Lean 'N Tasty, beef or pork	1 slice (.3 oz.)	10
BAKING POWDER, any type	Any quantity	0
BAMBOO SHOOTS	Any quantity	0
BANANA	Any quantity	0

Food and Description	Measure or Quantity	Cholesterol (milligrams)
BARLEY	Any quantity	0
BEAN, BLACK OR BROWN, dry	1 cup	0
BEAN & FRANKFURTER		
DINNER, frozen, Morton	10¾-oz. dinner	44
BEAN, GREEN		
Fresh	Any quantity	0
Frozen, Birds Eye		
Cut or French	⅓ of 9-oz. pkg.	0
French, with almonds	⅓ of 9-oz. pkg.	0
Whole, deluxe	⅓ of 9-oz. pkg.	0
BEAN, ITALIAN, frozen, Birds Eye	⅓ of 9-oz. pkg.	0
BEAN, KIDNEY OR RED, fresh or canned	Any quantity	0
BEAN, LIMA		
Raw or canned	Any quantity	0
Frozen, Birds Eye		
Baby	⅓ of 10-oz. pkg.	0
Baby butter	⅓ of 10-oz. pkg.	0
Fordhook	⅓ of 10-oz. pkg.	0
Tiny, deluxe	⅓ of 10-oz. pkg.	0
BEAN, MUNG, dry	Any quantity	0
BEAN, PINTO	Any quantity	0
BEAN SPROUT	Any quantity	0
BEAN, YELLOW OR WAX	Any quantity	0

BEEF. Values for beef cuts are given below for "lean and fat" and for "lean only." Beef purchased by the consumer at the retail store usually is trimmed to about one-half-inch layer of fat. This is the meat described as "lean and fat." If all the fat that can be cut off with a

Food and Description	Measure or Quantity	Cholesterol (milligrams)

knife is removed, the remainder is the "lean only." These cuts still contain flecks of fat known as "marbling" distributed through the meat. Cooked meats are medium done. Choice grade cuts

Brisket		
Raw, lean & fat	1 lb. (weighed with bone)	259
Raw, lean & fat	1 lb. (weighed without bone)	308
Raw, lean only	1 lb.	295
Braised		
Lean & fat	4 oz.	107
Lean only	4 oz.	103
Chuck		
Raw	1 lb. (weighed with bone)	259
Raw, lean & fat	1 lb. (weighed without bone)	308
Raw, lean only	1 lb.	295
Braised or pot-roasted		
Lean & fat	4 oz.	107
Lean only	4 oz.	103

Dried (see **BEEF, CHIPPED**)

Filet mignon. There is no data available on its composition. For dietary estimates, the data for sirloin steak, lean only, afford the closest approximation.

Flank		
Raw, 100% lean	1 lb.	295
Braised, 100% lean	4 oz.	103

Food and Description	Measure or Quantity	Cholesterol (milligrams)
Foreshank		
Raw, lean & fat	1 lb. (weighed with bone)	163
Simmered		
Lean & fat	4 oz.	107
Lean only	4 oz.	103
Ground		
Lean		
Raw	1 lb.	295
Raw	1 cup (8 oz.)	147
Broiled	4 oz.	103
Regular		
Raw	1 lb.	308
Raw	1 cup (8 oz.)	154
Broiled	4 oz.	107
Heel of round		
Raw, lean & fat	1 lb.	308
Raw, lean only	1 lb.	295
Roasted		
Lean & fat	4 oz.	107
Lean only	4 oz.	103
Hindshank		
Raw, lean & fat	1 lb. (weighed with bone)	142
Raw, lean & fat	1 lb. (weighed without bone)	308
Raw, lean only	1 lb.	295
Simmered		
Lean & fat	4 oz.	107
Lean only	4 oz.	103
Neck		
Raw, lean & fat	1 lb. (weighed with bone)	247

Food and Description	Measure or Quantity	Cholesterol (milligrams)
Pot-roasted		
Lean & fat	4 oz.	107
Lean only	4 oz.	103
Oxtail, raw	1 lb. (weighed with bone)	73
Plate		
Raw, lean & fat	1 lb. (weighed with bone)	275
Raw, lean only	1 lb.	295
Simmered		
Lean & fat	4 oz.	107
Lean only	4 oz.	103
Rib roast		
Raw, lean & fat	1 lb. (weighed with bone)	284
Raw, lean only	1 lb.	295
Roasted		
Lean & fat	4 oz.	107
Lean only	4 oz.	103
Lean only, chopped	1 cup (4.5 oz.)	130
Round		
Raw, lean & fat	1 lb. (weighed with bone)	299
Raw, lean only	1 lb.	295
Broiled		
Lean & fat	4 oz.	107
Lean only	4 oz.	103
Rump		
Raw, lean & fat	1 lb. (weighed with bone)	262
Raw, lean only	1 lb.	295
Roasted		
Lean & fat	4 oz.	107

Food and Description	Measure or Quantity	Cholesterol (milligrams)
Lean only	4 oz.	103
Steak, club		
Raw, lean & fat	1 lb. (weighed with bone)	259
Raw, lean & fat	1 lb. (weighed without bone)	308
Raw, lean only	1 lb.	295
Broiled		
Lean & fat	4 oz.	107
Lean only	4 oz.	103
One 8-oz. steak (weighed without bone before cooking) will give you		
Lean & fat	5.9 oz.	156
Lean only	3.4 oz.	87
Steak, porterhouse		
Raw	1 lb. (weighed with bone)	281
Broiled		
Lean & fat	4 oz.	107
Lean only	4 oz.	103
One 16-oz. steak (weighed with bone before cooking) will give you		
Lean & fat	10.2 oz.	271
Lean only	5.9 oz.	151
Steak, ribeye, broiled		
One 10-oz. steak (weighed before cooking without bone) will give you		
Lean & fat	7.3 oz.	195
Lean only	3.8 oz.	97
Steak, sirloin, double-bone		

Food and Description	Measure or Quantity	Cholesterol (milligrams)
Raw, lean & fat	1 lb. (weighed without bone)	308
Raw, lean & fat	1 lb. (weighed with bone)	253
Raw, lean only	1 lb.	295
Broiled		
Lean & fat	4 oz.	107
Lean only	4 oz.	103
One 16-oz. steak (weighed before cooking with bone) will give you		
Lean & fat	8.9 oz.	237
Lean only	5.9 oz.	151
One 12-oz. steak (weighed with bone before cooking) will give you		
Lean & fat	6.6 oz.	177
Lean only	4.4 oz.	113
Steak, sirloin, hipbone		
Raw, lean & fat	1 lb. (weighed with bone)	262
Raw, lean only	1 lb.	295
Broiled		
Lean & fat	4 oz.	107
Lean only	4 oz.	103
Steak, sirloin, wedge & round-bone		
Raw, lean & fat	1 lb. (weighed with bone)	287
Raw, lean only	1 lb.	295
Broiled		
Lean & fat	4 oz.	107
Lean only	4 oz.	103

Food and Description	Measure or Quantity	Cholesterol (milligrams)
Steak, T-bone		
Raw, lean & fat	1 lb. (weighed with bone)	275
Broiled		
Lean & fat	4 oz.	107
Lean only	4 oz.	103
One 16-oz. steak (weighed before cooking with bone) will give you		
Lean & fat	9.8 oz.	261
Lean only	5.5 oz.	142
BEEF, CHIPPED		
Cooked, home recipe, creamed	½ cup (4.3 oz.)	33
Frozen, creamed, Morton	5-oz. pkg.	17
BEEF DINNER or ENTREE, frozen		
Morton, Regular		
Dinner	10-oz. dinner	66
Entree, patty	5-oz. pkg.	35
Country Table, sliced	14-oz. dinner	87
Steak House		
Chopped sirloin	9½-oz. dinner	134
Rib eye	9-oz. dinner	134
Sirloin strip	9½-oz. dinner	134
Tenderloin	9½-oz. dinner	134
Stouffer's Lean Cuisine, oriental	8⅝-oz. pkg.	35
BEEF PIE, frozen, Morton	8-oz. pie	40
BEEF STEW		
Home recipe, made with lean beef chuck	1 cup (8.6 oz.)	64
Canned, regular pack	1 cup (8.6 oz.)	34
Frozen, Morton, Family Meal	2-lb. pkg.	200
BEER & ALE	Any quantity	0

Food and Description	Measure or Quantity	Cholesterol (milligrams)
BEET	Any quantity	0
BIG H, burger sauce, Hellmann's	1 T. (.5 oz.)	4
BIG WHEEL, Hostess	1 piece (1 ⅓ oz.)	7
BLACKBERRY	Any quantity	0
BLACKBERRY JELLY	Any quantity	0
BLACK-EYED PEAS, fresh, canned, or frozen	Any quantity	0
BLINTZ, frozen, King Kold, cheese	2½-oz. piece	8
BLUEBERRY, fresh, canned, or frozen	Any quantity	0
BLUEBERRY PRESERVE OR JAM	Any quantity	0
BOLOGNA, Oscar Mayer		
Beef	.8-oz. slice	13
Beef	1-oz. slice	16
Beef	1.3-oz. slice	22
Meat	.8-oz. slice	13
Meat	1-oz. slice	17
Meat	1.3-oz. slice	22
Meat	2-oz. slice	34
BOLOGNA & CHEESE, Oscar Mayer	.8-oz. slice	14
BOYSENBERRY	Any quantity	0
BOYSENBERRY JELLY	Any quantity	0
BRAINS, all animals, raw	4 oz.	2268
BRAN	Any quantity	0
BRAN BREAKFAST CEREAL	Any quantity	0
BRAUNSCHWEIGER, Oscar Mayer, chub	1 oz.	39
BRAZIL NUT	Any quantity	0
BREAD		
Bran, Arnold, Bran'nola	1.2-oz. slice	0

Food and Description	Measure or Quantity	Cholesterol (milligrams)
Cracked wheat, Wonder	1-oz. slice	Tr.
French		
Arnold, Francisco	¹⁄₁₆ of loaf (1 oz.)	0
Wonder	1-oz. slice	0
Hillbilly	1-oz. slice	Tr.
Hollywood		
Dark	1-oz. slice	Tr.
Light	1-oz. slice	Tr.
Honey wheatberry, Arnold	1.2-oz. slice	3
Low-sodium, Wonder	1-oz. slice	Tr.
Pumpernickel		
Arnold	1-oz. slice	0
Levy's	1.1-oz. slice	0
Raisin		
Arnold tea	.9-oz. slice	3
Thomas' cinnamon	.8-oz. slice	0
Roman Meal	1-oz. slice	Tr.
Rye		
Arnold		
Dill	1-oz. slice	0
Jewish	1.1-oz. slice	3
Melba Thin	.7-oz. slice	0
Levy's, real	1-oz. slice	0
Wonder	1-oz. slice	Tr.
7-Grain, Home Pride	1-oz. slice	Tr.
Sourdough, Di Carlo	1-oz. slice	0
Sprouted wheat, Arnold	.9-oz. slice	<5
Wheat (See also Cracked Wheat or Whole Wheat)		
Arnold, Bran'nola, hearty	1.3-oz. slice	<5
Fresh Horizons	1-oz. slice	0
Fresh & Natural	1-oz. slice	0

Food and Description	Measure or Quantity	Cholesterol (milligrams)
Home Pride	1-oz. slice	Tr.
Wonder, family	1-oz. slice	Tr.
Wheatberry, Home Pride		
Honey	1-oz. slice	Tr.
Regular	1-oz. slice	0
White		
Arnold		
Bran'nola	1.3-oz. slice	0
Brick Oven	.8-oz. slice	<5
Brick Oven	1.1-oz. slice	<5
Country	1.2-oz. slice	<5
Heartstone	1.1-oz. slice	0
Measure Up	.5-oz. slice	<5
Fresh Horizons	1-oz. slice	0
Home Pride	1-oz. slice	Tr.
Wonder		
Regular	1-oz. slice	Tr.
Buttermilk	1-oz. slice	Tr.
Whole wheat		
Arnold		
Brick Oven	.8-oz. slice	<5
Measure Up	.5-oz. slice	<5
Stone ground	.8-oz. slice	0
Home Pride	1-oz. slice	Tr.
Thomas' 100%	.8-oz. slice	0
Wonder 100%	1-oz. slice	Tr.
*BREAD DOUGH, frozen Rich's		
French, Italian, wheat, or white	½0 of loaf	0
Raisin	½0 of loaf	3
BREAD PUDDING, with raisins, home recipe	1 cup (9.3 oz.)	170
BROCCOLI		
Raw	Any quantity	0

Food and Description	Measure or Quantity	Cholesterol (milligrams)
Boiled	Any quantity	0
Frozen, Birds Eye		
With almonds & selected		
seasonings	⅓ of 10-oz. pkg.	0
In cheese	⅓ of 10-oz. pkg.	4
Chopped, cuts, or florets	⅓ of 10-oz. pkg.	0
Spears		
Regular	⅓ of 10-oz. pkg.	0
In butter sauce	⅓ of 10-oz. pkg.	8
Deluxe	⅓ of 10-oz. pkg.	0
& water chestnuts with selected		
seasonings	⅓ of 10-oz. pkg.	0
BRUSSELS SPROUT		
Raw, trimmed	1 lb.	0
Boiled, drained	3-4 sprouts	0
Frozen, Birds Eye		
Regular	⅓ of 10-oz. pkg.	0
In butter sauce	⅓ of 10-oz. pkg.	5
Baby, with cheese sauce	⅓ of 10-oz. pkg.	4
Baby, deluxe	⅓ of 10-oz. pkg.	0
BUCKWHEAT, groats, Pocono		
Brown, whole	1 oz.	Tr.
Cracked, brown, & white	1 oz.	Tr.
White, whole	1 oz.	Tr.
BULGUR (from hard red winter wheat)		
Dry	1 lb.	0
Canned, unseasoned	4-oz. serving	0
BURGUNDY WINE	Any quantity	0
BURGUNDY WINE, SPARKLING	Any quantity	0
BUTTER, salted or unsalted		
Regular	¼ lb.	284
Regular	1 T. (.5 oz.)	34

Food and Description	Measure or Quantity	Cholesterol (milligrams)
Regular	1 pat (5 grams)	12
Breakstone	1 T.	29
Whipped	1 T. (9 grams)	22
Whipped	1 stick (2.7 oz.)	190
BUTTERSCOTCH MORSELS,		
Nestlé's	1 oz.	1

C

Food and Description	Measure or Quantity	Cholesterol (milligrams)
CABBAGE, white or red, fresh or canned	Any quantity	0
CAKE		
Angel food, home recipe	1/12 of 8″ cake	0
Carrot, Hostess	3-oz. piece	77
Chocolate, home recipe, with chocolate icing, 2-layer	1/12 of 9″ cake	43
Crumb, Hostess	1¼-oz. piece	11
Devil's food, home recipe, with chocolate icing, 2-layer	1/16 of 9″ cake	32
Fruit, home recipe, dark	1/30 of 8″ loaf	7
Fruit loaf, Hostess	½ of 5-oz. cake	3
Honey, Holland Honey Cake, low-sodium		
Fruit and raisin	½″ slice (.9 oz.)	0

Food and Description	Measure or Quantity	Cholesterol (milligrams)
Orange and premium unsalted	½" slice (.9 oz.)	0
Sponge, home recipe	¹⁄₁₂ of 10" cake	162
Yellow, home recipe, made with butter, with chocolate icing, 2-layer	¹⁄₁₆ of 9" cake	33
Frozen, cheesecake		
Morton, Great Little Desserts		
Cherry	6-oz. cake	106
Cream cheese	6-oz. cake	116
Pineapple	6-oz. cake	106
Strawberry	6-oz. cake	106
Rich's Viennese	¹⁄₁₄ of 42-oz. cake	25
CAKE ICING, Duncan Hines, chocolate, regular, fudge, or milk or vanilla	¹⁄₁₂ of can	7
CAKE MIX		
Regular		
Angel Food, Duncan Hines	¹⁄₁₂ of pkg.	0
*Cheesecake, Jell-O	⅛ of cake	28
Devil's food, Duncan Hines, deluxe	¹⁄₁₂ of pkg.	0
Yellow, Duncan Hines, deluxe	¹⁄₁₂ of pkg.	0
*Dietetic, Dia-Mel; Estee	¹⁄₁₀ of cake	0
CANDY. The following values of candies from the U.S. Department of Agriculture are representative of the types sold commercially. These values may be useful when individual brands or sizes are not known:		
Almond, sugar-coated or Jordan	1 oz.	0

Food and Description	Measure or Quantity	Cholesterol (milligrams)
Candy corn	1 oz.	0
Gum drops	1 oz.	0
CANDY, REGULAR		
Baby Ruth	1.8-oz. piece	0
Butterfinger	1.6-oz. bar	0
Caramel, Caramel Nip, Pearson	1 piece	0
Chocolate bar, Nestlé		
Crunch	1⅟₁₆-oz. bar	6
Milk	.35-oz. bar	2
Milk	1⅟₁₆-oz. bar	7
Chocolate bar with almonds, Nestlé	1-oz.	7
Chocolate Parfait, Pearson	1 piece (6.5 grams)	0
Licorice Nips, Pearson	1 piece (6.5 grams)	0
Mint Parfait, Pearson	1 piece (6.5 grams)	0
Peanut brittle, Planters, Jumbo Peanut Block Bar	1 oz.	0
Peanut butter cup, Reese's	.6-oz. cup	2
Reggie Bar	2-oz. bar	0
CANDY, DIETETIC		
Carob bar, Joan's Natural		
Coconut	3-oz. bar	27
Fruit & nut	3-oz. bar	26
Honey bran	3-oz. bar	26
Peanut	3-oz. bar	24
Chocolate or chocolate-flavored bar, Estee		
Coconut, fruit & nut, milk, or toasted bran	.2-oz. square	1
Crunch	.2-oz. square	1
Estee-ets, with peanuts, Estee	1 piece (1.4 grams)	Tr.
Gum drops, Estee, any flavor	1 piece (1.8 grams)	0
Hard candy		
Estee, assorted fruit	1 piece (.1 oz.)	0

Food and Description	Measure or Quantity	Cholesterol (milligrams)
Louis Sherry	1 piece (.1 oz.)	0
Lollipop, Estee; Louis Sherry	1 piece (.2 oz.)	0
Mint, Estee	1 piece (1.1 grams)	0
Peanut butter cup, Estee	1 cup (.3 oz.)	Tr.
Raisins, chocolate-covered, Estee	1 piece (1.2 grams)	Tr.
T.V. Mix, Estee	1 piece (1.6 grams)	Tr.
CANNELLONI, frozen, Stouffer's		
Beef & pork with mornay sauce	9⅝-oz. pkg.	50
Cheese with tomato sauce	9⅛-oz. pkg.	45
CANTALOUPE, fresh	Any quantity	0
CARROT, raw or canned	Any quantity	0
CASABA MELON	Any quantity	0
CASHEW NUT, raw or roasted	Any quantity	0
CATSUP	Any quantity	0
CAULIFLOWER		
Raw	Any quantity	0
Boiled flowerbuds, drained	½ cup (2.2 oz.)	0
Frozen, Birds Eye		
Regular or florets, deluxe	⅓ of 10-oz. pkg.	0
With almonds & selected seasonings	⅓ of 10-oz. pkg.	0
With cheese sauce	⅓ of 10-oz. pkg.	4
CAVIAR, STURGEON, whole eggs	1 T. (.6 oz.)	748
CELERIAC ROOT, raw	Any quantity	0
CELERY, all varieties	Any quantity	0
CHABLIS WINE	Any quantity	0
CHEESE		
American or cheddar		
Regular	1 oz.	25
Cube, natural	1″ cube (.6 oz.)	17
Featherweight, low-sodium	1 oz.	30
Fisher	1 oz.	30
Laughing Cow, natural	1 oz.	28
Sargento		

Food and Description	Measure or Quantity	Cholesterol (milligrams)
Crock, sharp	1 oz.	18
Midget, regular or sharp, sliced or sticks	1 oz.	30
Shredded, non-dairy	1 oz.	2
Blue		
Natural	1 oz.	24
Sargento, cold pack or crumbled	1 oz.	21
Bonbino, Laughing Cow, natural	1 oz.	27
Brick		
Natural	1 oz.	26
Sargento, sliced	1 oz.	27
Brie, Sargento, Danish Danko	1 oz.	21
Burgercheese, Sargento, Danish Danko	1 oz.	27
Camembert		
Domestic	1 oz.	26
Sargento, Danish Danko	1 oz.	17
Colby		
Natural	1 oz.	27
Fisher	1 oz.	33
Sargento, shredded or sliced	1 oz.	27
Cottage, unflavored	½ cup (4.3 oz.)	23
Cream, plain, unwhipped	1 oz.	31
Edam		
Natural	1 oz.	29
Sargento	1 oz.	25
Farmers, Sargento	1 oz.	16
Feta, Sargento, Danish, cups	1 oz.	25
Gouda		
Laughing Cow	1 oz.	28
Sargento, baby, caraway, or smoked	1 oz.	32
Wispride	1 oz.	24
Gruyere, Swiss Knight	1 oz.	24

Food and Description	Measure or Quantity	Cholesterol (milligrams)
Havarti, Sargento		
Creamy	1 oz.	21
Creamy, 60% mild	1 oz.	21
Hot pepper, Sargento, sliced	1 oz.	27
Jarlsberg, Sargento, Norwegian	1 oz.	16
Kettle Moraine, Sargento	1 oz.	9
Limburger, Sargento, natural	1 oz.	26
Mozzarella		
Fisher, part skim milk	1 oz.	19
Sargento		
Bar, rounds, shredded regular or with spices, sliced for pizza, or square	1 oz.	15
Whole milk	1 oz.	22
Muenster		
Natural	1 oz.	25
Sargento, red rind	1 oz.	27
Wispride	1 oz.	26
Neufchatel, natural	1 oz.	22
Nibblin Curds, Sargento	1 oz.	30
Parmesan		
Natural	1 oz.	27
Sargento, wedge	1 oz.	19
Pizza, Sargento, shredded or sliced, non-dairy	1 oz.	2
Pot, Sargento, regular, French onion or garlic	1 oz.	0
Provolone		
Natural	1 oz.	28
Sargento, sliced	1 oz.	20
Ricotta		
Natural		
Whole milk	1 oz.	14
Part skim milk	1 oz.	9

Food and Description	Measure or Quantity	Cholesterol (milligrams)
Sargento		
Part skim milk	1 oz.	9
Whole milk	1 oz.	14
Romano, Sargento, wedge	1 oz.	29
Samsoe, Sargento, Danish	1 oz.	24
Semisoft, Laughing Cow		
Babybel		
Regular	1 oz.	22
Mini	¾ oz.	18
Bonbel		
Regular	1 oz.	24
Mini	¾ oz.	18
Reduced calorie	1 oz.	11
String, Sargento	1 oz.	15
Swiss		
domestic, natural, or process	1 oz.	28
Fisher, natural	1 oz.	27
Sargento, domestic or Finland, sliced	1 oz.	26
CHEESE FONDUE, Swiss Knight	1 oz.	14
CHEESE FOOD		
American or cheddar		
Process	1 oz.	20
Fisher, Ched-O-Mate or Sandwich-Mate	1 oz.	5
Sargento	1 oz.	18
Weight Watchers, colored or white	1-oz. slice	8
Wispride		
Hickory smoked	1 oz.	20
& port wine	1 oz.	20
Cheez-ola, Fisher	1 oz.	Tr.
Chef's Delight, Fisher	1 oz.	6

Food and Description	Measure or Quantity	Cholesterol (milligrams)
Count Down, Fisher	1 oz.	Tr.
Cracker snack, Sargento	1 oz.	27
Pizza-Mate, Fisher	1 oz.	Tr.
CHEESE SPREAD		
American or cheddar		
Fisher	1 oz.	21
Laughing Cow	1 oz.	18
Gruyere, Laughing Cow, La Vache		
Que Rit	1 oz.	18
Pimiento, Price	1 oz.	15
Provolone, Laughing Cow	1 oz.	18
Velveeta, Kraft	1 oz.	20
CHEESE STRAW, made with lard	5″ × ⅜″ × ⅜″ piece (6 grams)	2
CHENIN BLANC WINE, Louis M.		
Martini, 12½% alcohol	Any quantity	0
CHERRY, fresh, sour, or sweet	Any quantity	0
CHERRY, CANDIED	1 oz.	0
CHERRY, MARASCHINO	1 oz. (with liq.)	0
CHERRY PRESERVES OR JAM		
Sweetened, Smucker's	1 T. (.7 oz.)	0
Dietetic, Louis Sherry	1 T. (.6 oz.)	0
CHESTNUT	Any quantity	0
CHEWING GUM		
Sweetened, Big Red; Doublemint; Freedent; Hubba Bubba; Juicy Fruit, Spearmint, Wrigley's; Teaberry	1 stick	Tr.
Dietetic, Orbit, Wrigley's	1 piece	Tr.
CHICKEN		
Broiler, cooked, meat only	4 oz.	99
Capon, raw, with bone	1 lb. (weighed ready-to-cook)	325

Food and Description	Measure or Quantity	Cholesterol (milligrams)
Capon, raw, meat & skin	4 oz.	92
Fryer		
Raw		
Ready-to-cook	1 lb. (weighed with bone)	310
Meat & skin	1 lb.	367
Meat only	1 lb.	358
Dark meat & skin	1 lb.	399
Light meat & skin	1 lb.	304
Dark meat without skin	1 lb.	399
Light meat without skin	1 lb.	358
Back	1 lb. (weighed with bone)	198
Breast	1 lb. (weighed with bone)	239
Leg or drumstick	1 lb. (weighed with bone)	239
Neck	1 lb. (weighed with bone)	177
Thigh	1 lb. (weighed with bone)	275
Wing	1 lb. (weighed with bone)	180
Fried. A 2½-lb. chicken (weighed before cooking with bone) will give you		
Back	1 back (2.2 oz.)	35
Breast	½ breast (3⅓ oz.)	61
Leg or drumstick	1 leg (2 oz.)	34
Neck	1 neck (2.1 oz.)	37
Rib	1 rib (.7 oz.)	12
Thigh	1 thigh (2¼ oz.)	44
Wing	1 wing (1¾ oz.)	25

Food and Description	Measure or Quantity	Cholesterol (milligrams)
Hen and cock		
Raw		
Ready-to-cook	1 lb. (weighed ready-to-cook)	324
Meat & skin	1 lb.	367
Meat only	1 lb.	445
Dark meat without skin	1 lb.	399
Light meat without skin	1 lb.	304
Stewed		
Meat & skin	4 oz.	91
Meat only	4 oz.	99
Chopped	½ cup (2.5 oz.)	63
Diced	½ cup (2.4 oz.)	59
Ground	½ cup (2 oz.)	49
Roaster		
Raw	1 lb. (weighed with bones)	325
Meat & skin with giblets	1 lb.	445
Meat & skin	1 lb.	445
Meat only	1 lb.	367
Dark meat without skin	1 lb.	399
White meat without skin	1 lb.	304
Roasted		
Total edible	4 oz.	99
Meat & skin with giblets	4 oz.	92
Meat & skin	4 oz.	99
Meat only	4 oz.	99
Dark meat without skin	4 oz.	99
Light meat without skin	4 oz.	99
CHICKEN A LA KING		
Home recipe	1 cup (8.6 oz.)	186
Frozen, Morton	5-oz. pkg.	27
CHICKEN DINNER OR ENTREE, frozen		

Food and Description	Measure or Quantity	Cholesterol (milligrams)
Morton		
Regular		
Boneless	10-oz. dinner	48
Fried	11-oz. dinner	85
Sliced	5-oz. pkg.	27
Country Table, fried	15-oz. entree	98
King Size, fried		
Dinner	17-oz. dinner	141
Entree	12-oz. entree	128
Stouffer's Lean Cuisine		
Glazed with vegetable rice	8½-oz. serving	55
& vegetables with vermicelli	12¾-oz. serving	40
CHICKEN FRICASSEE, home recipe	1 cup (8.5 oz.)	96
CHICKEN, FRIED, frozen, Morton		
Assorted	2-lb. pkg.	470
Breast portion	22-oz. pkg.	316
CHICKEN GIZZARD		
Raw	4 oz.	164
Simmered	4 oz.	221
CHICKEN PIE, frozen		
USDA	8-oz. pie	29
Morton	8-oz. pie	36
CHICK-FIL-A, sandwich	5.4-oz. serving	55
CHICK PEAS OR GARBANZOS, dry	Any quantity	0
CHILI SAUCE	Any quantity	0
CHIVES, raw	1 T. (3 grams)	0
CHOCO-DILE, Hostess	2-oz. piece	20
CHOCOLATE, BAKING		
Baker's		
Bitter or unsweetened	1 oz. square	Tr.
Semi-sweet		

Food and Description	Measure or Quantity	Cholesterol (milligrams)
Regular	1-oz. square	Tr.
Chips	¼ cup (1½ oz.)	Tr.
Sweetened, German's	1 oz. square	Tr.
Hershey's		
Bitter or unsweetened	1 oz.	0
Sweetened		
Dark chips, regular or mini	1 oz.	0
Milk, chips	1 oz.	0
Nestlé		
Bitter or unsweetened, Choco-bake	1-oz. packet	0
Sweet or semi-sweet, morsels	1 oz.	5
CHOCOLATE, HOT, home recipe	1 cup (8.8 oz.)	31
CHOP SUEY		
Home recipe, with meat	1 cup (8.8 oz.)	64
Canned, with meat	4 oz.	3
CHOW MEIN		
Canned, La Choy		
Regular		
Beef	¾ cup	<20
Beef pepper oriental	¾ cup	<20
Chicken	¾ cup	<20
Meatless	¾ cup	Tr.
Shrimp	¾ cup	<50
*Bi-pack		
Beef	¾ cup	<20
Beef pepper oriental or shrimp	¾ cup	<20
Chicken	¾ cup	<20
Pork	¾ cup	<10
Vegetable	¾ cup	<10
Frozen, Stouffer's Lean Cuisine,		

Food and Description	Measure or Quantity	Cholesterol (milligrams)
chicken, with rice	11 ¼-oz. serving	25
CHOW MEIN SEASONING MIX,		
Kikkoman	1 ⅛-oz. pkg.	Tr.
CLAM		
Raw		
All kinds, meat only	4 med. clams (3 oz.)	42
Hard or round, meat only	1 cup (8 oz.)	114
Soft, meat only	1 cup (8 oz.)	114
Canned, meat only	½ cup (2.8 oz.)	50
CLAM JUICE, Snow	½ cup	13
CLARET WINE, Taylor, 12.5% alcohol	3 fl. oz.	0
COCOA		
Dry, unsweetened		
Low-fat	1 T. (5 grams)	0
High-fat	1 T. (5 grams)	0
Mix, regular		
Alba '66, instant, all flavors	1 envelope	Tr.
Hershey's		
Hot	1 oz.	0
Instant	3 T. (.75 oz.)	0
Nestlé, with or without mini marshmallows	1 oz.	0
COCONUT		
Fresh	Any quantity	0
Dried, canned, or packaged		
Baker's		
Angel Flake		
Packaged in bag	⅓ cup (.9 oz.)	Tr.
Canned	⅓ cup (.9 oz.)	Tr.
Cookie cut	⅓ cup (1.3 oz.)	Tr.
Premium shred	⅓ cup (1 oz.)	Tr.
Southern style	⅓ cup (.9 oz.)	Tr.

Food and Description	Measure or Quantity	Cholesterol (milligrams)
COD		
Raw, whole	1 lb. (weighed whole)	70
Raw, meat only	4 oz.	57
Dehydrated, lightly salted	4 oz.	93
COFFEE	Any quantity	0
COFFEE SOUTHERN	1 fl. oz.	0
COLD DUCK WINE, Great Western, pink, 12% alcohol	3 fl. oz.	0
COLLARDS, fresh, canned, or frozen	Any quantity	0
COOKIE, REGULAR		
Brownie, Hostess		
Large	2-oz. piece	17
Small	1¼-oz. piece	11
Ladyfinger	3¼″ × 1⅜″ × 1⅛″ (.4 oz.)	40
Waffle creme, Dutch Twins	1 piece (.3 oz.)	0
COOKIE, DIETETIC, Estee		
Chocolate chip	1 piece	<5
Coconut or lemon thin	1 piece	0
Sandwich duplex	1 piece (.3 oz.)	0
Vanilla, thin	1 piece (.2 oz.)	0
Wafer, chocolate covered	1 piece (.9 oz.)	<5
*COOKIE DOUGH, frozen, Rich's		
Chocolate chip	1 cookie	7
Oatmeal	1 cookie	1
Oatmeal & raisins	1 cookie	6
Peanut butter	1 cookie	2
Sugar	1 cookie	6
COOKIE, HOME RECIPE, brownie with nuts	1¾″ × 1¾″ × ⅞″	17

Food and Description	Measure or Quantity	Cholesterol (milligrams)
COOKIE MIX, regular, Duncan Hines	1 piece	0
COOKING SPRAY, Mazola No Stick	2-second spray	0
CORIANDER SEED, French's	1 tsp. (1.4 grams)	0
CORN		
Fresh or canned	Any quantity	0
Frozen, Birds Eye		
On the cob	Any quantity	0
Whole kernel	⅓ of 10-oz. pkg.	0
With butter sauce	⅓ of 10-oz. pkg.	4
CORNBREAD		
Home recipe		
Southern style, prepared with degermed cornmeal	2½″ × 2½″ × 1⅝″ piece	58
Southern style, prepared with whole-ground cornmeal	4 oz.	79
*Mix	2½″ × 2½″ × 1⅜″ piece	38
*CORN DOGS, frozen, Oscar Mayer	1 piece (4 oz.)	38
CORNED BEEF, packaged, Oscar Mayer	1-oz. slice	13
CORN FLAKES, cereal	Any quantity	0
CORNMEAL, WHITE or **YELLOW**	Any quantity	0
CORN PUDDING, home recipe	1 cup (8.6 oz.)	103
COWPEA	Any quantity	0
CRAB		
Fresh, steamed		
Whole	½ lb. (weighed in shell)	218

Food and Description	Measure or Quantity	Cholesterol (milligrams)
Meat only	4 oz.	113
Canned, drained	4 oz.	115
CRAB APPLE, flesh only	¼ lb.	0
CRAB, DEVILED, home recipe	4 oz.	116
CRAB IMPERIAL, home recipe	1 cup (7.8 oz.)	308
CRACKER, PUFFS, & CHIPS		
Bacon Nips	1 oz.	0
Cheetos, crunchy or puffy	1 oz.	0
Cheez Balls, Planters	1 oz.	0
Cheez Curls, Planters	1 oz.	0
Roman Meal Wafer, boxed	1 piece	Tr.
Tortilla chips, Doritos, nacho or taco	1 oz.	0
Unsalted, Estee	1 piece (.1 oz.)	Tr.
Wheat wafer, Estee, 6 Calorie	1 piece	3
CRANAPPLE JUICE, Ocean Spray	Any quantity	0
CRANBERRY, fresh	Any quantity	0
CRANBERRY-ORANGE RELISH, uncooked	Any quantity	0
CRANBERRY SAUCE, home recipe or canned	Any quantity	0
CREAM		
Half & Half	1 T. (.5 oz.)	6
Light, table or coffee	1 T. (.5 oz.)	10
Light, whipping	1 T. (.5 oz.)	3
Heavy whipping	1 T. (.5 oz.)	20
Sour	1 T. (.5 oz.)	8
Sour, imitation, Pet	1 T. (.5 oz.)	Tr.
Substitute (See **CREAM SUBSTITUTE**)		
CREAM PUFFS		
Home recipe, custard filling	3½″ × 2″ piece (4.6 oz.)	187

Food and Description	Measure or Quantity	Cholesterol (milligrams)
Frozen, Rich's, Bavarian or chocolate	1⅓-oz. piece	23
CREAM SUBSTITUTE		
Coffee Rich, Rich's	½ oz.	0
Cremora	1 tsp. (2 grams)	2
CUCUMBER	Any quantity	0
CUPCAKE, Hostess		
Chocolate	1 cupcake (1¾ oz.)	5
Orange	1 cupcake (1½ oz.)	13
CURRANT	Any quantity	0
CUSTARD		
Home recipe, baked	½ cup (4.7 oz.)	139
Chilled, Swiss Miss, chocolate or egg flavor	4-oz. container	3

D

Food and Description	Measure or Quantity	Cholesterol (milligrams)
DAIRY QUEEN/BRAZIER		
Banana split	13.5-oz. serving	30
Brownie Delight, hot fudge	9.4-oz. serving	26
Buster Bar	5¼-oz. piece	7
Chicken sandwich	7.8-oz. sandwich	77
Cone		
Plain, any flavor		
Small	3-oz. cone	9
Regular	5-oz. cone	14
Large	7½-oz. cone	21
Dipped, chocolate		
Small	3¼-oz. cone	9
Regular	5½-oz. cone	16
Large	8¼-oz. cone	23
Dilly Bar	3-oz. piece	8
Double Delight	9-oz. serving	26

Food and Description	Measure or Quantity	Cholesterol (milligrams)
DQ Sandwich	2.1-oz. sandwich	39
Fish sandwich		
Plain	6-oz. sandwich	60
With cheese	6¼-oz. sandwich	71
Float	14-oz. serving	20
Freeze, vanilla	12-oz. serving	20
French fries		
Regular	2½-oz. serving	11
Large	4-oz. serving	17
Frozen dessert	4-oz. serving	11
Hamburger		
Plain		
Single	5.2-oz. burger	45
Double	7.4-oz. burger	85
Triple	9.6-oz. burger	135
With cheese		
Single	5.7-oz. burger	50
Double	8.4-oz. burger	95
Triple	10.63-oz. burger	145
Hot dog		
Regular		
Plain	3.5-oz. serving	45
With cheese	4-oz. serving	55
With chili	4½-oz. serving	55
Super		
Plain	6.2-oz. serving	80
With cheese	6.9-oz. serving	100
With chili	7.7-oz. serving	100
Malt, chocolate		
Small	10¼-oz. serving	35
Regular	14¾-oz. serving	50
Large	20¾-oz. serving	70
Mr. Misty		
Plain		

Food and Description	Measure or Quantity	Cholesterol (milligrams)
Small	8¼-oz. serving	0
Regular	11.64-oz. serving	0
Large	15½-oz. serving	0
Kiss	3.14-oz. serving	0
Float	14.5-oz. serving	20
Freeze	14.5-oz. serving	30
Onion rings	3-oz. serving	15
Parfait	10-oz. serving	30
Peanut Butter Parfait	10¾-oz. serving	30
Shake, chocolate		
Small	10¼-oz. serving	35
Regular	14¾-oz. serving	50
Large	20¾-oz. serving	70
Strawberry shortcake	11-oz. serving	25
Sundae, chocolate		
Small	3¾-oz. serving	10
Regular	6¼-oz. serving	20
Large	8¾-oz. serving	30
Tomato	½ oz.	0
DANDELION GREENS, raw	Any quantity	0
DATE	Any quantity	0
DESSERT CUPS, Hostess	¾-oz. piece	9
DING DONG, Hostess	1 cake (1⅓ oz.)	7
DINNER, FROZEN See individual listings such as **BEEF, CHICKEN, TURKEY**		
DIP		
Blue cheese, Breakstone	1 oz.	14
Jalapeño, Hain, natural	1 oz.	0
Onion bean, Hain, natural	1 oz.	0
DISTILLED LIQUOR, any brand	Any quantity	0
DOUGHNUT		
Regular, Hostess		
Chocolate-coated	1-oz. piece	4

Food and Description	Measure or Quantity	Cholesterol (milligrams)
Cinnamon	1-oz. piece	6
Donettes		
Frosted	1 piece	5
Powdered	1 piece	2
Krunch	1-oz. piece	4
Old fashioned		
Plain	1.5-oz. piece	10
Glazed	2-oz. piece	11
Plain	1-oz. piece	7
Powdered	1-oz. piece	7
Frozen, Morton		
Regular		
Bavarian creme	2-oz. piece	11
Boston creme	2⅓-oz. piece	11
Chocolate-iced	1.5-oz. piece	10
Glazed	1.5-oz. piece	10
Jelly	1.8-oz. piece	11
Mini	1.1-oz. piece	13
Donut Holes	⅕ of 7¾-oz. pkg.	5
Morning Light		
Chocolate	2-oz. piece	6
Glazed	2-oz. piece	6
Jelly	2.6-oz. piece	8

E

Food and Description	Measure or Quantity	Cholesterol (milligrams)
ECLAIR, frozen, Rich's, chocolate	1 piece (2.6 oz.)	60
EGG, CHICKEN		
Raw		
White only	1 large egg (1.2 oz.)	0
White only	1 cup (9 oz.)	0
Yolk only	1 large egg (.6 oz.)	250
Yolk only	1 cup (8.5 oz.)	3552
Whole, small	1 egg (1.3 oz.)	186
Whole, medium	1 egg (1.5 oz.)	220
Whole, large	1 egg (1.8 oz.)	251
Whole	1 cup (8.8 oz.)	1265
Whole, extra large	1 egg (2 oz.)	289
Whole, jumbo	1 egg (2.3 oz.)	325
Cooked		

Food and Description	Measure or Quantity	Cholesterol (milligrams)
Boiled	1 large egg (1.8 oz.)	251
Poached	1 large egg	242
Scrambled, mixed with milk & cooked in fat	1 large egg	263
Scrambled, mixed with milk & cooked in fat	1 cup (7.8 oz.)	904
Dried		
Whole	1 cup (3.8 oz.)	2052
Yolk	1 cup (3.4 oz.)	2525
EGGPLANT	Any quantity	0
EGG SUBSTITUTE		
Egg Magic, Featherweight	½ of envelope	15
Eggstra, Tillie Lewis	1 lg. egg substitute	70
*Scramblers, Morningstar Farms	1 egg substitute	0
Second Nature, Avoset	3 T.	0
ELDERBERRY, fresh	Any quantity	0
ENCHILADA OR ENCHILADA DINNER, frozen, beef, Morton	11-oz. dinner	18
ENDIVE, CURLY, raw	Any quantity	0

F

Food and Description	Measure or Quantity	Cholesterol (milligrams)
FARINA	Any quantity	0
FAT, COOKING	Any quantity	0
FENNEL SEED	1 tsp. (2.1 grams)	0
FIG	Any quantity	0
FILBERT	Any quantity	0
FISH DINNER, frozen		
Morton	9-oz. dinner	74
Stouffer's Lean Cuisine		
Filet, divan	12⅜-oz. pkg.	85
Florentine	9-oz. pkg.	100
FIT'N FROSTY, Alba '77		
Chocolate	¾-oz. envelope	1
Strawberry	¾-oz. envelope	1
Vanilla	¾-oz. envelope	Tr.

Food and Description	Measure or Quantity	Cholesterol (milligrams)
FLOUNDER, raw		
Whole	1 lb. (weighed whole)	75
Meat only	4 oz.	57
FLOUR, any type	Any quantity	0
FRANKFURTER, raw or cooked		
Meat	1 frankfurter (10 per lb.)	29
Oscar Mayer		
Beef		
Regular	1.6-oz. frankfurter	27
Jumbo	2-oz. frankfurter	35
Big One	4-oz. frankfurter	69
Little Wiener	2″ frankfurter	5
Wiener	1.2-oz. frankfurter	18
Wiener	1.6-oz. frankfurter	24
Wiener	2-oz. frankfurter	30
Wiener	2.7-oz. frankfurter	40
Wiener	4-oz. frankfurter	60
Wiener, with cheese	1.6-oz. frankfurter	31
FRITTERS, home recipe, clam	2″ × 1¾″ (1.4 oz.)	52
FROG LEGS, raw		
Bone-in	1 lb. (weighed with bone)	147
Meat only	4 oz.	57
FROZEN DESSERT, dietetic, Baskin-Robbins, Special Diet		
Mountain Coffee	1 scoop (2½ fl. oz.)	2
Sunny Orange	1 scoop (2½ fl. oz.)	Tr.
Wild Strawberry	1 scoop (2½ fl. oz.)	Tr.

Food and Description	Measure or Quantity	Cholesterol (milligrams)
FRUIT COCKTAIL	Any quantity	0
*FRUIT PUNCH,** mix, dietetic, Crystal Light	6 fl. oz.	0
FRUIT SALAD, canned	Any quantity	0

G

Food and Description	Measure or Quantity	Cholesterol (milligrams)
GARLIC	Any quantity	0
GELATIN, unflavored dry	7-gram envelope	0
GELATIN DESSERT, canned or mix	Any quantity	0
GIN, unflavored (See **DISTILLED LIQUOR**)		
***GINGERBREAD MIX**	⅑ of 8″ square	Tr.
GOOSEBERRY	Any quantity	0
GRAPE, fresh or canned	Any quantity	0
GRAPEFRUIT, fresh or canned	Any quantity	0
GRAPEFRUIT JUICE	Any quantity	0
GRAPE NUTS, cereal, Post	Any quantity	0
GRAVY WITH MEAT OR TURKEY, frozen, Morton, Family Meal		
Gravy, mushroom, & beef patty	¼ of 2-lb. pkg.	54

Food and Description	Measure or Quantity	Cholesterol (milligrams)
Gravy, onion, & beef patty	¼ of 2-lb. pkg.	54
& beef, sliced	¼ of 2-lb. pkg.	71
& salisbury steak	¼ of 2-lb. pkg.	55
& turkey croquettes	¼ of 2-lb. pkg.	42
& turkey, sliced	¼ of 2-lb. pkg.	38
GUAVA, COMMON, fresh	Any quantity	0
GUAVA, STRAWBERRY, fresh	Any quantity	0

H

Food and Description	Measure or Quantity	Cholesterol (milligrams)
HADDOCK, raw, meat only	4 oz.	68
HALIBUT		
Raw		
Whole	1 lb. (weighed whole)	134
Meat only	4 oz.	57
Broiled	4″ × 3″ × ½″ steak (4.4 oz.)	75
HAM (See also **PORK**)		
Canned, Oscar Mayer, Jubilee, extra lean, cooked	1-oz. serving	12
Packaged, Oscar Mayer		
Chopped	1-oz. slice	14
Cooked, smoked	1-oz. slice	14
Jubilee, boneless		
Sliced	8-oz. slice	112

Food and Description	Measure or Quantity	Cholesterol (milligrams)
Steak, 95% fat free	2-oz. steak	26
HAM & CHEESE, packaged, Oscar Mayer loaf	1-oz. slice	16
HAM DINNER, frozen, Morton	10-oz. dinner	64
HEADCHEESE, Oscar Mayer	1 oz.	25
HEART		
Beef		
Lean, raw	1 lb.	680
Lean, braised	4 oz.	311
Lean, braised, chopped, or diced	1 cup (5.1 oz.)	397
Chicken		
Raw	1 lb.	771
Simmered	1 heart (5 grams)	12
Simmered, chopped, or diced	1 cup (5.1 oz.)	335
Turkey		
Raw	1 lb.	680
Simmered	4 oz.	270
Simmered, chopped, or diced	1 cup (5.1 oz.)	345
HERRING, raw, Atlantic		
Whole	1 lb. (weighed whole)	197
Meat only	4 oz.	96
HICKORY NUT	Any quantity	0
HO-HO, Hostess	1-oz. piece	13
HOMINY GRITS		
Dry		
Degermed	1 oz.	0
Degermed	½ cup (2.8 oz.)	0
Pocono, creamy	1 oz.	Tr.
Cooked, degermed	⅔ cup (5.6 oz.)	0
HONEY, strained	Any quantity	0
HONEYCOMB, cereal, Post		
Regular	1⅓ cups (1 oz.)	0
Strawberry	1⅓ cups (1 oz.)	Tr.

Food and Description	Measure or Quantity	Cholesterol (milligrams)
HONEYDEW, fresh	Any quantity	0
HORSERADISH	Any quantity	0
HOSTESS O'S, Hostess	2¼-oz. piece	14
HYACINTH BEAN	Any quantity	0

I

Food and Description	Measure or Quantity	Cholesterol (milligrams)
ICE CREAM and **FROZEN CUSTARD,** with salt added		
10% fat, regular ice cream	3-fl.-oz. container	20
10% fat, regular ice cream	1 cup (4.7 oz.)	53
10% fat, frozen custard or French ice cream	1 cup (4.7 oz.)	97
10% fat, frozen custard or French ice cream	3-fl.-oz. container	36
16% fat, rich ice cream	1 cup (5.2 oz.)	84
ICE MILK		
Hardened	1 cup (4.6 oz.)	26
Soft-serv	1 cup (6.3 oz.)	35
IRISH WHISKEY (See **DISTILLED LIQUOR)**		

J

Food and Description	Measure or Quantity	Cholesterol (milligrams)
JACKFRUIT, fresh	Any quantity	0
JAM, sweetened	Any quantity	0
JELL-O FRUIT & CREAM BAR	1.7-oz. bar	5
JELL-O GELATIN POPS	Any quantity	0
JELL-O PUDDING POPS	2-oz. piece	1
JELLY, sweetened	Any quantity	0
JERUSALEM ARTICHOKE	Any quantity	0
JUJUBE or **CHINESE DATE**	Any quantity	0

K

Food and Description	Measure or Quantity	Cholesterol (milligrams)
KALE	Any quantity	0
KIDNEY		
Beef, raw	4 oz.	425
Beef, braised	4 oz.	912
Calf, raw	4 oz.	425
Hog, raw	4 oz.	425
Lamb, raw	4 oz.	425
KOHLRABI	Any quantity	0
*KOOL-AID, General Foods	Any quantity	0
KUMQUAT, fresh	Any quantity	0

L

Food and Description	Measure or Quantity	Cholesterol (milligrams)
LAKE COUNTRY WINE, Taylor	Any quantity	0
LAMB, choice grade		
Chop, broiled		
Loin. One 5-oz. chop (weighed before cooking with bone) will give you		
Lean & fat	2.8 oz.	76
Lean only	2.3 oz.	65
Rib. One 5-oz. chop (weighed before cooking with bone) will give you		
Lean & fat	2.9 oz.	80
Lean only	2 oz.	56
Leg		
Raw, lean & fat	1 lb. (weighed with bone)	271

Food and Description	Measure or Quantity	Cholesterol (milligrams)
Roasted, lean & fat	4 oz.	111
Roasted, lean only	4 oz.	113
Shoulder		
Raw, lean & fat	1 lb. (weighed with bone)	274
Roasted, lean & fat	4 oz.	111
Roasted, lean only	4 oz.	113
LAMB'S QUARTERS	Any quantity	0
LARD	1 cup (7.2 oz.)	195
	1 T. (.5 oz.)	12
LASAGNA, frozen, Stouffer's Lean Cuisine, zucchini	11 oz. serving	20
LEEKS, raw	Any quantity	0
LEMON	Any quantity	0
LEMONADE, canned or frozen, Country Time	Any quantity	0
LEMON JUICE, fresh	Any quantity	0
*****LEMON-LIMEADE DRINK,** mix, dietetic, Crystal Light	6 fl. oz.	0
LENTIL	Any quantity	0
LETTUCE, any type	Any quantity	0
LIL' ANGELS, Hostess	1-oz. piece	2
LIME, fresh, peeled fruit	Any quantity	0
LITCHI NUT	Any quantity	0
LIVER		
Beef		
Raw	1 lb.	1361
Fried	4 oz.	497
Calf		
Raw	1 lb.	1361
Fried	4 oz.	497
Chicken		
Raw	1 lb.	2517
Simmered	4 oz.	846

Food and Description	Measure or Quantity	Cholesterol (milligrams)
Hog		
Raw	1 lb.	1361
Fried	4 oz.	497
Lamb		
Raw	1 lb.	1361
Braised	4 oz.	497
Turkey		
Raw	1 lb.	1973
Simmered	4 oz.	679
LOBSTER,		
Raw, meat only	4 oz.	96
Cooked, meat only	1 cup (5.1 oz.)	123
LOBSTER NEWBERG, home recipe	1 cup (8.8 oz.)	455
LOGANBERRY	Any quantity	0
LONGAN	Any quantity	0
LOQUAT, fresh, flesh only	Any quantity	0
LUNCHEON MEAT, Oscar Mayer (See also individual listings such as **BOLOGNA, HAM**)		
All meat	1-oz. slice	16
Bar-B-Que Loaf, 90% fat free	1-oz. slice	11
Ham & cheese (See **HAM & CHEESE**)		
Ham roll sausage, Oscar Mayer	1-oz. slice	13
Honey loaf, 95% fat free	1-oz. slice	11
Liver cheese	1.3-oz. slice	69
Luxury loaf	1-oz. slice	11
New England Brand Sliced sausage	.8-oz. slice	14
Old fashioned loaf	1-oz. slice	14
Olive loaf	1-oz. slice	11

Food and Description	Measure or Quantity	Cholesterol (milligrams)
Peppered loaf	1-oz. slice	14
Pickle & pimiento loaf	1-oz. slice	11
Picnic loaf	1-oz. slice	12

M

Food and Description	Measure or Quantity	Cholesterol (milligrams)
MACADAMIA NUT	Any quantity	0
MACARONI, dry	Any quantity	0
MACARONI & CHEESE		
Home recipe, baked	1 cup (7.1 oz.)	42
Frozen, Morton		
Casserole	8-oz. casserole	24
Dinner	11-oz. dinner	18
Family Meal	2-lb. pkg.	88
MACKEREL, Atlantic		
Raw		
Whole	1 lb. (weighed whole)	233
Meat only	4 oz.	108
Broiled with vegetable shortening	8½″ × 2½″ × ½″ fillet (3.7 oz.)	106

Food and Description	Measure or Quantity	Cholesterol (milligrams)
Canned, solids & liq.	4 oz.	107
MALT, dry	1 oz.	0
MANGO, fresh	Any quantity	0
MANHATTAN COCKTAIL,		
National Distillers, 20% alcohol	3 fl. oz.	0
MARGARINE		
Salted		
Made with liquid oil, regular	Any quantity	0
Made with two-thirds animal fat & one-third vegetable fat		
	1 lb.	227
	4 oz. (1 stick)	57
	1 cup or 1 tub (8 oz.)	113
	1 T. (⅛ of stick .5 oz.)	7
	1 pat (1″ × ⅓″ × 1″, 5 grams)	2
Unsalted		
Made with hydrogenated fats, regular or soft	Any quantity	0
Made with liquid oil, regular or soft	Any quantity	0
	1 lb.	0
	4 oz. (1 stick)	0
	1 cup or 1 tub (8 oz.)	0
	1 T. (⅛ stick, .5 oz.)	0
	1 T. (⅛ stick, .5 oz.)	0
	1 pat (1″ × ⅓″ × 1″, 5 grams)	0

Food and Description	Measure or Quantity	Cholesterol (milligrams)
Made with two-thirds animal fat & one-third vegetable fat		
	1 lb.	227
	4 oz. (1 stick)	57
	1 cup or 1 tub (8 oz.)	113
	1 T. (⅛ stick, .5 oz.)	7
	1 pat (1″ × ⅓″ × 1″, 5 grams)	0
MARGARITA COCKTAIL, National Distillers, 12½% alcohol	3 fl. oz.	0
MARINADE MIX, Kikkoman	1-oz. pkg.	0
MARMALADE, sweetened	Any quantity	0
MARSHMALLOW FLUFF	1 heaping tsp.	0
MAYONNAISE		
Real, Hellmann's, Best Foods	1 T. (.5 oz.)	7
Imitation or dietetic, Weight Watchers	1 T.	5
MAYPO, cereal	Any quantity	0
McDONALD'S		
Big Mac	1 hamburger	86
Cheeseburger	1 cheeseburger	37
Chicken McNuggets	1 serving	76
Chicken McNuggets Sauce		
Barbecue	1.1-oz. serving	Tr.
Honey	.5-oz. serving	Tr.
Hot mustard	1.1-oz. serving	3
Sweet & sour	1.1-oz. serving	Tr.
Cookies		
Chocolate chip	1 package	18

Food and Description	Measure or Quantity	Cholesterol (milligrams)
McDonaldland	1 package	10
Egg McMuffin	1 serving	229
Egg, scrambled	1 serving	349
English muffin, with butter	1 muffin	13
Filet-O-Fish	1 sandwich	47
Hamburger	1 hamburger	25
Hot cakes with butter & syrup	1 serving	47
Potato		
Fried	Regular order	8
Hash brown	2-oz. serving	7
Quarter Pounder		
Regular	5.9-oz. serving	67
With cheese	6.8-oz. serving	96
Sausage	1.9-oz. serving	43
Shakes		
Chocolate	10.3-oz. serving	30
Strawberry	10.2-oz. serving	32
Vanilla	10.3-oz. serving	31
Sundae		
Caramel	5.8-oz. serving	26
Hot fudge	5.8-oz. serving	18
Strawberry	5.8-oz. serving	20
MEATBALL STEW, frozen, Stouffer's Lean Cuisine	10-oz. pkg.	65
MEAT LOAF DINNER, frozen, Morton		
Regular	11-oz. dinner	61
Family Meal, & tomato sauce	1-lb. pkg.	212
MEAT TENDERIZER, Adolph's	1 tsp.	0
MEXICAN DINNER, frozen, Morton	11-oz. dinner	16
MILK, CONDENSED, sweetened, canned	1 T. (.7 oz.)	6
MILK, DRY, whole, packed cup	1 cup (5.1 oz.)	158

Food and Description	Measure or Quantity	Cholesterol (milligrams)
MILK, EVAPORATED, canned		
Regular		
Unsweetened	1 cup (8.9 oz.)	79
Carnation	1 cup (8.9 oz.)	62
Skimmed, Carnation	1 cup (9 oz.)	2
MILK, FRESH		
Whole, 3.5% fat	1 cup (8.6 oz.)	34
Skim	1 cup (8.6 oz.)	5
Buttermilk, cultured, fresh	1 cup (8.6 oz.)	5
Chocolate milk drink, fresh		
With whole milk	1 cup (8.8 oz.)	32
With skim milk & 2% added		
butterfat	1 cup (8.8 oz.)	20
MOLASSES	Any quantity	0
MUFFIN		
Blueberry		
Hostess	1¾-oz. muffin	15
Morton		
Regular	1.6-oz. muffin	9
Rounds	1.5-oz. muffin	14
Bran, Arnold, Bran'nola	2.3-oz. muffin	0
Corn, Morton	1.7-oz. muffin	14
English		
Arnold, extra crisp	2.3-oz. muffin	Tr.
Roman Meal	2.3-oz. muffin	Tr.
Thomas' raisin	2.2-oz. muffin	0
Wonder	2-oz. muffin	0
Plain, home recipe	1.4-oz. muffin	21
Raisin		
Arnold	2½-oz. muffin	0
Wonder	2-oz. muffin	0
Sourdough, Wonder	2-oz. muffin	0
MUFFIN MIX, bran, Duncan Hines	¹⁄₁₂ of pkg.	0
MUSHROOM, raw	Any quantity	0

Food and Description	Measure or Quantity	Cholesterol (milligrams)
MUSTARD, prepared	Any quantity	0
MUSTARD GREENS		
Raw, whole	1 lb. (weighed untrimmed)	0
Frozen, chopped, Birds Eye	⅓ of 10-oz. pkg.	0
MUSTARD SPINACH	Any quantity	0

N

Food and Description	Measure or Quantity	Cholesterol (milligrams)
NECTARINE, fresh	Any quantity	0
NEW ZEALAND SPINACH	Any quantity	0
NOODLE		
Dry	1 oz.	27
Dry, 1½″ strips	1 cup (2.6 oz.)	67
Cooked	1 oz.	9
NOODLE, CHOW MEIN	½ cup (1 oz.)	2
NUT, MIXED, Planters oil or dry roasted	Any quantity	0

O

Food and Description	Measure or Quantity	Cholesterol (milligrams)
OAT FLAKES, cereal, Post	⅔ cup (1 oz.)	0
OATMEAL, dry	½ cup (1.2 oz.)	0
OIL, SALAD OR COOKING	Any quantity	0
OKRA		
Raw, whole	1 lb. (weighed untrimmed)	0
Frozen, Birds Eye, whole, baby, or cut	⅓ of 10-oz. pkg.	0
OLIVE	Any quantity	0
ONION		
Raw	Any quantity	0
Boiled, drained	Any quantity	0
Dehydrated, flakes or powder	Any quantity	0
Frozen, Birds Eye		
Chopped or small, whole	Any quantity	0
Small, with cream sauce	⅓ of 9-oz. pkg.	Tr.

Food and Description	Measure or Quantity	Cholesterol (milligrams)
ONION, GREEN, raw	Any quantity	0
ONION, WELCH, raw	Any quantity	0
ORANGE, fresh	Any quantity	0
*ORANGE DRINK MIX, dietetic Crystal Light	Any quantity	0
ORANGE JUICE, fresh, canned, or frozen	Any quantity	0
ORANGE PEEL, CANDIED	1 oz.	0
OVEN FRY, General Foods	Any quantity	0
OYSTER		
Raw		
Eastern, meat only	19–31 small or 13–19 med.	120
Pacific & Western, meat only	6–9 small or 4–6 med. (8.5 oz.)	120
Canned, shelled, whole, solids & liq.	1 cup (8.5 oz.)	51
OYSTER STEW, home recipe		
1 part oysters to 2 parts milk by volume	1 cup (8.5 oz.)	62
1 part oysters to 3 parts milk by volume	1 cup (8.5 oz.)	58

P

Food and Description	Measure or Quantity	Cholesterol (milligrams)
*PANCAKE & WAFFLE MIX		
Plain, made with milk & egg	4″ pancake	54
Dietetic, Dia-Mel	3″ pancake	0
PAPAW, fresh	Any quantity	0
PAPAYA, fresh	Any quantity	0
PARSLEY, fresh	Any quantity	0
PARSNIP	Any quantity	0
PASSION FRUIT, fresh	Any quantity	0
PASTRY SHELL, home recipe, baked, made with vegetable shortening	1 shell (1.5 oz.)	0
PDQ		
Chocolate or strawberry	1 T. (.6 oz.)	0
Egg Nog	2 heaping T. (1 oz.)	Tr.
PEA, green		
Raw or canned	Any quantity	0

Food and Description	Measure or Quantity	Cholesterol (milligrams)
Frozen, Birds Eye		
Regular	⅓ of 10-oz. pkg.	0
In butter sauce	⅓ of 10-oz. pkg.	5
In cream sauce	⅓ of 8-oz. pkg.	1
Tiny, tender, deluxe	⅓ of 10-oz. pkg.	0
PEA & CARROT, frozen, Birds Eye	⅓ of 10-oz. pkg.	0
PEA, CROWDER, frozen, Birds Eye	⅕ of 16-oz. pkg.	0
PEA, MATURE SEED, dry	Any quantity	0
PEA POD	Any quantity	0
PEACH, fresh, canned, or frozen	Any quantity	0
PEACH NECTAR, canned	6 fl. oz.	0
PEANUT, raw or roasted	Any quantity	0
PEANUT BUTTER	Any quantity	0
PEAR	Any quantity	0
PEBBLES, cereal, Post	Any quantity	0
PECAN, raw or roasted	Any quantity	0
PECTIN, FRUIT, Certo or Sure-Jell	Any quantity	0
PEPPER, black	Any quantity	0
PEPPER, CHILI, raw or canned, green	Any quantity	0
PEPPER, STUFFED, home recipe, with beef & crumbs	2¾" × 2½" pepper with 1⅛ cups stuffing	56
PERSIMMON	Any quantity	0
PICKLE, cucumber, fresh, bread & butter; dill, sour, or sweet	Any quantity	0
PIE		
Regular, non-frozen		
Apple, Hostess	4½-oz. pie	19
Berry, Hostess	4½-oz. pie	19
Blueberry, Hostess	4½-oz. pie	19

Food and Description	Measure or Quantity	Cholesterol (milligrams)
Cherry, Hostess	4½-oz. pie	19
Custard, home recipe	⅙ of 9″ pie	160
Lemon, Hostess	4½-oz. pie	32
Lemon chiffon, home recipe, made with lard	⅙ of 9″ pie	183
Lemon meringue, home recipe, made with lard	⅙ of 9″ pie	130
Peach, Hostess	4½-oz. pie	19
Pineapple, home recipe, 1 crust, made with lard	⅙ of 9″ pie	93
Strawberry, Hostess	¼-oz. pie	13
Frozen, Morton		
Apple		
Regular	⅙ of 24-oz. pie	12
Great Little Desserts		
Regular	8-oz. pie	23
Dutch	7¾-oz. pie	13
Banana cream		
Regular	⅙ of 14-oz. pie	9
Great Little Desserts	3½-oz. pie	15
Blueberry		
Great Little Desserts	8-oz. pie	23
Regular	⅙ of 24-oz. pie	12
Cherry		
Regular	⅙ of 24-oz. pie	12
Great Little Desserts	8-oz. pie	23
Chocolate	⅙ of 14-oz. pie	9
Chocolate cream, Great Little Desserts	3½-oz. pie	15
Coconut cream, Great Little Desserts	3½-oz. pie	15
Coconut custard, Great Little Desserts	6½-oz. pie	110
Lemon	⅙ of 14-oz. pie	9

Food and Description	*Measure or Quantity*	*Cholesterol (milligrams)*
Lemon cream, Great Little Desserts	3½-oz. pie	15
Mince	⅙ of 24-oz. pie	12
Peach		
Regular	⅙ of 24-oz. pie	12
Great Little Desserts	8-oz. pie	22
Pumpkin	⅙ of 24-oz. pie	44
Strawberry cream, Banquet	⅙ of 14-oz. pie	168
PIGEON PEA	Any quantity	0
PIMIENTO, canned	Any quantity	0
PINEAPPLE, fresh	Any quantity	0
PINEAPPLE & GRAPEFRUIT JUICE DRINK, canned	Any quantity	0
PINEAPPLE JUICE, canned	Any quantity	0
PINEAPPLE-ORANGE JUICE, canned	6 fl. oz.	0
PINE NUT	Any quantity	0
PISTACHIO NUT	Any quantity	0
PITANGA, fresh	Any quantity	0
PIZZA PIE MIX, Ragú, Pizza Quick		
Crust only	1/12 of pkg.	0
*Pizza	¼ of pie	25
PIZZA SAUCE, Ragú, Pizza Quick, regular or chunky	Any quantity	0
PLANTAIN, raw	Any quantity	0
PLUM	Any quantity	0
POMEGRANATE, raw	Any quantity	0
PONDEROSA RESTAURANT		
Beef, chopped, patty only, raw		
Regular	3½ oz.	67
Big	4.8-oz.	94
Double Deluxe	5.9 oz.	116

Food and Description	Measure or Quantity	Cholesterol (milligrams)
Junior, Square Shooter	1.6 oz.	31
Steakhouse Deluxe	2.96 oz.	58
Beverages, milk		
Regular	8 fl. oz.	34
Chocolate	8 fl. oz.	33
Bun, hot dog	1 bun	15
Chicken strips, raw		
Adult portion	2¾ oz.	60
Children's portion	1.4 oz.	30
Filet Mignon, raw	3.8 oz. (edible portion)	70
Filet of sole, fish only	3-oz. piece	59
Fish, baked, before baking	4.9-oz. serving	98
Ham & cheese		
Cheese, Swiss	2 slices (.8 oz.)	19
Ham	2½ oz.	35
Hot dog, child's, meat only	1.6-oz. hot dog	35
New York strip steak	6.1 oz. (edible portion)	122
Prime ribs, raw		
Regular	4.2 oz. (edible portion)	83
Imperial	8.4 oz. (edible portion)	165
King	6 oz. (edible portion)	118
Pudding		
Butterscotch	4½ oz.	3
Chocolate	4½ oz.	15
Vanilla	4½ oz.	16
Ribeye, raw	3.2 oz. (edible portion)	56
Ribeye & Shrimp, raw		

Food and Description	Measure or Quantity	Cholesterol (milligrams)
Ribeye	3.2 oz.	56
Shrimp	2.2 oz.	56
Roll, kaiser	2.2-oz. roll	77
Shrimp dinner, raw	7 pieces (3½ oz.)	122
Sirloin, raw		
Regular	3.3 oz. (edible portion)	66
Super	6½ oz. (edible portion)	128
Tips	4 oz. (edible portion)	74
T-bone, raw	4.3 oz. (edible portion)	85
Topping, whipped	¼ oz.	5
POPOVER, home recipe	2¾" at top (1.4 oz.)	59
PORK, medium-fat		
Fresh		
Boston butt		
Raw	1 lb. (weighed with bone & skin)	264
Roasted, lean & fat	4 oz.	101
Roasted, lean only	4 oz.	100
Chop		
Broiled, lean & fat	1 chop (4 oz., weighed with bone)	67
Broiled, lean & fat	1 chop (4 oz., weighed with bone)	76
Broiled, lean & fat	1 chop (3 oz., weighed without bone)	75

Food and Description	Measure or Quantity	Cholesterol (milligrams)
Ham (See Also **HAM**)		
Raw	1 lb. (weighed with bone & skin)	239
Roasted, lean & fat	4 oz.	101
Roasted, lean only	4 oz.	100
Loin		
Raw	1 lb. (weighed with bone)	221
Roasted, lean & fat	4 oz.	101
Roasted, lean only	4 oz.	100
Picnic		
Raw	1 lb. (weighed with bone & skin)	231
Simmered, lean & fat	4 oz.	101
Simmered, lean only	4 oz.	100
Spareribs		
Raw, with bone	1 lb. (weighed with bone)	169
Raw, without bone	1 lb. (weighed with bone)	281
Braised, lean & fat	4 oz.	101
PORK RINDS, Baken-Ets	1-oz. serving	6
PORT WINE, Great Western, 18% alcohol	Any quantity	0
*POSTUM, instant, regular or coffee-flavored	6 fl. oz.	0
POTATO		
Raw	Any quantity	0
Cooked		
Au gratin, with cheese	½ cup (4.3 oz.)	18
Baked, peeled, no salt added	2½″ dia. potato (3.5 oz.)	0
Boiled, peeled before boiling, no salt	4.3-oz. potato	0

Food and Description	Measure or Quantity	Cholesterol (milligrams)
Canned, solids & liq.	Any quantity	0
Frozen, Birds Eye		
Cottage fries	2.8-oz. serving	0
Crinkle cuts		
Regular	3-oz. serving	0
Deep Gold	3-oz. serving	0
Farm style wedge	3-oz. serving	0
French fries		
Regular	3-oz. serving	0
Deep Gold	3-oz. serving	0
Hash browns		
Regular	4-oz. serving	0
Shredded	¼ of 12-oz. pkg.	0
Shoestring	3-oz. serving	0
Steak fries	3-oz. serving	0
Tasti Fries	2½-oz. serving	0
Tasti Puffs	¼ of 10-oz. pkg.	32
Tiny Taters	⅕ of 16-oz. pkg.	0
Triangles	1½ oz. serving	0
Whole, peeled	3.2 oz. serving	0
POTATO CHIP, Lay's or Pringle's	Any quantity	0
POTATO SALAD, home recipe, with mayonnaise & French dressing, hard-cooked eggs, seasonings	½ cup (4.4 oz.)	81
PRETZEL	Any quantity	0
PRICKLY PEAR, fresh	Any quantity	0
PRUNE JUICE	Any quantity	0
PUDDING OR PIE FILLING		
Home recipe		
Rice, made with raisins	½ cup (4.7 oz.)	15
Tapioca cream	½ cup (2.9 oz.)	80
Frozen, Rich's	Any quantity	0

Food and Description	Measure or Quantity	Cholesterol (milligrams)
*Mix, sweetened, regular &		
Instant		
Banana		
Jell-O, cream		
Regular	½ cup	18
Instant	½ cup	16
Royal		
Regular	½ cup	14
Instant	½ cup	15
Butter pecan, Jello-O, instant	½ cup	16
Butterscotch		
Jell-O		
Regular	½ cup	16
Instant	½ cup	16
Royal		
Regular	½ cup	14
Instant	½ cup	15
Chocolate		
Jell-O		
Plain		
Regular	½ cup	16
Instant	½ cup	16
Fudge		
Regular	½ cup	17
Instant	½ cup	17
Milk		
Regular	½ cup	17
Instant	½ cup	17
My-T-Fine, regular	½ cup	169
Coconut		
Jell-O cream		
Regular	½ cup	18
Instant	½ cup	17
Royal, instant	½ cup	15

Food and Description	Measure or Quantity	Cholesterol (milligrams)
Custard		
Jell-O Americana	½ cup	81
Royal, Regular	½ cup	14
Flan, Royal, regular	½ cup	14
Lemon		
Jell-O		
Regular	½ cup	93
Instant	½ cup	13
Royal, instant	½ cup	15
Pineapple, Jell-O, cream, instant	½ cup	16
Pistachio, Jell-O, instant	½ cup	17
Tapioca		
Jell-O Americana		
Chocolate	½ cup	16
Vanilla	½ cup	16
Royal, vanilla	½ cup	14
Vanilla		
Jell-O		
Plain, instant	½ cup	17
French, regular	½ cup	16
Royal	½ cup	15
*Mix, dietetic		
Butterscotch		
Dia-Mel	½ cup	2
D-Zerta	½ cup	3
Estee	½ cup	2
Chocolate		
Dia-Mel	½ cup	2
D-Zerta	½ cup (4.6 oz.)	3
Estee	½ cup	2
Louis Sherry	½ cup (4.2 oz.)	2
Lemon		
Dia-Mel	½ cup (4.2 oz.)	0
Estee	½ cup	2

Food and Description	Measure or Quantity	Cholesterol (milligrams)
Vanilla		
Dia-Mel	½ cup (4.2 oz.)	2
D-Zerta	½ cup	2
Estee	½ cup	2
PUFFED RICE	Any quantity	0
PUFFED WHEAT	Any quantity	0
PUFF, VANILLA, frozen, Rich's	1.8-oz. piece	40
PUMPKIN, fresh or canned	Any quantity	0
PUMPKIN SEED, dry	Any quantity	0

Q

Food and Description	Measure or Quantity	Cholesterol (milligrams)
QUIK, Nestlé	Any quantity	0
QUINCE, fresh	Any quantity	0

R

Food and Description	Measure or Quantity	Cholesterol (milligrams)
RABBIT, domesticated		
Raw, meat only	4 oz.	74
Stewed, meat only	4 oz.	103
RADISH	Any quantity	0
RASPBERRY, black or red	Any quantity	0
RASPBERRY PRESERVE OR JAM	1 T.	0
RELISH, sour or sweet	Any quantity	0
RHINE WINE, Great Western, 12% alcohol	3 fl. oz.	0
RHUBARB	Any quantity	0
*RICE, raw	Any quantity	0
RICE BRAN	1 oz.	0
RICE, FRIED, (See also **RICE MIX**), frozen, Birds Eye	3.7-oz. serving	Tr.
RICE, FRIED, SEASONING MIX,		

Food and Description	Measure or Quantity	Cholesterol (milligrams)
Kikkoman	1-oz. pkg.	Tr.
*RICE MIX, Minute Rice		
Beef, rib roast	½ cup (4.1 oz.)	10
Chicken, drumstick	½ cup (3.8 oz.)	11
Fried	½ cup (3.4 oz.)	0
Long grain & wild	½ cup (4.1 oz.)	10
Spanish	½ cup (5.2 oz.)	11
RICE, SPANISH, frozen, Birds Eye	3.7-oz. serving	0
RICE & VEGETABLE, frozen, Birds Eye		
French style	3.7-oz. serving	0
Peas with mushrooms	2⅓ oz. serving	0
RICE WINE		
Chinese, 20.7% alcohol	1 fl. oz.	38
Japanese, 10.6% alcohol	1 fl. oz.	72
ROE, raw, Salmon, sturgeon, or turbot	4 oz.	401
ROLL OR BUN		
Commercial type, non-frozen		
Biscuit, Wonder	1¼-oz. piece	<2
Brown & Serve, Wonder	1-oz. piece	Tr.
Dinner		
Home Pride	1-oz. piece	Tr.
Wonder	1¼-oz. piece	<2
Dinner party rounds, Arnold	.7-oz. piece	3
Frankfurter		
Arnold Hot Dog	1.3-oz. piece	0
Wonder	2-oz. piece	Tr.
French, Arnold, Francisco		
Regular	2-oz. roll	0
Sourdough	1.1-oz. piece	0
Hamburger		
Arnold	1.4-oz. piece	0
Wonder	2-oz. piece	0

Food and Description	Measure or Quantity	Cholesterol (milligrams)
Hoggie, Wonder	6-oz. piece	<8
Honey, Hostess, glazed	3¾-oz. piece	23
Kaiser, Wonder	6-oz. piece	<8
Pan, Wonder	1¼-oz. piece	Tr.
Sandwich, Arnold		
Francisco	2-oz. piece	0
Soft, plain, or with poppy		
seed	1.3-oz. piece	<5
Soft with sesame seeds	1.3-oz. piece	<5
Frozen, honey, Morton		
Regular	2.3-oz. piece	0
Mini	1.3-oz. piece	0
*ROLL OR BUN DOUGH, frozen, Rich's		
Cinnamon	2¼-oz. piece	4
Danish, round	1 piece	25
Hamburger, regular	1 piece	0
Parkerhouse	1 piece	0
ROMAN MEAL CEREAL, 2- or 5-minute	⅓ cup (1 oz.)	Tr.
ROSE WINE, Great Western, 12% alcohol	3 fl. oz.	0
RUTABAGA, raw or boiled	Any quantity	0
RYE, whole grain	1 oz.	0

S

Food and Description	Measure or Quantity	Cholesterol (milligrams)
SAFFLOWER SEED, in hull	Any quantity	0
SALAD DRESSING		
Regular		
Bleu or blue cheese, Wish-Bone, chunky	1 T.	1
Boiled, home recipe	1 T. (.6 oz.)	12
Caesar, Wish-Bone	1 T.	Tr.
Cheddar & bacon, Wish-Bone	1 T. (.5 oz.)	Tr.
French, Wish-Bone	1 T.	0
Green Goddess, Wish-Bone	1 T.	Tr.
Italian, Wish-Bone	1 T.	0
Mayonnaise-type	1 T.	8
Russian, Wish-Bone	1 T.	0
Sour cream & bacon, Wish-Bone	1 T.	Tr.
Spin Blend, Hellmann's	1 T. (.6 oz.)	8

Food and Description	Measure or Quantity	Cholesterol (milligrams)
Thousand Island, Wish-Bone		
Regular	1 T.	5
Southern recipe		
Plain	1 T.	10
Bacon	1 T.	5
Dietetic or low-calorie		
Bleu or blue cheese		
Dia-Mel	1 T. (.5 oz.)	2
Walden Farms, chunky	1 T.	6
Wish-Bone, chunky	1 T.	Tr.
Buttermilk, Wish-Bone	1 T.	Tr.
Caesar, Estee, garlic	1 T. (.5 oz.)	0
Cucumber		
Dia-Mel, creamy	1 T. (.5 oz.)	0
Wish-Bone, creamy	1 T.	0
French		
Dia-Mel	1 T. (.5 oz.)	0
Walden Farms	1 T.	2
Wish-Bone		
Regular	1 T.	0
Sweet & spicy	1 T.	0
Garlic, Dia-Mel	1 T. (.5 oz.)	0
Herb garden, Estee	1 T.	0
Italian		
Dia-Mel, regular or creamy	1 T. (.5 oz.)	0
Estee, spicy	1 T.	0
Walden Farms		
Regular or low-sodium	1 T.	0
No sugar added	1 T.	0
Weight Watchers	1 T.	6
Wish-Bone, regular or creamy	1 T.	0
Onion & chive, Wish-Bone	1 T.	0
Onion & cucumber, Estee	1 T. (.5 oz.)	0
Red wine/vinegar, Dia-Mel	1 T.	0

Food and Description	Measure or Quantity	Cholesterol (milligrams)
Russian		
Weight Watchers	1 T.	6
Wish-Bone	1 T. (.5 oz.)	0
Thousand Island		
Dia-Mel	1 T.	5
Walden Farms	1 T.	8
Weight Watchers	1 T.	6
Wish-Bone	1 T.	5
Whipped, Dia-Mel	1 T.	2
Yogurt-buttermilk, Dia-Mel	1 T.	7
SALAD DRESSING MIX		
*Regular, Good Seasons		
Blue cheese	1 T. (.6 oz.)	Tr.
Buttermilk, farm style	1 T. (.6 oz.)	5
Classic herb	1 T.	0
Farm style	1 T.	4
French, old-fashioned	1 T.	0
Garlic, cheese	1 T.	Tr.
Garlic & herb	1 T.	0
Italian		
Regular, mild, or zesty	1 T. (.6 oz.)	0
Cheese	1 T. (.6 oz.)	Tr.
Tomato & herb	1 T. (.6 oz.)	0
*Dietetic, Italian, Good Seasons		
Regular	1 T.	0
Lite	1 T.	Tr.
SALAMI, Oscar Mayer		
For beer		
Regular	.8-oz. slice	13
Beef	.8-oz. slice	14
Cotto		
Regular	.8-oz. slice	14
Regular	1-oz. slice	18
Beef	.5-oz. slice	9

Food and Description	Measure or Quantity	Cholesterol (milligrams)
Beef	.8-oz. slice	14
Hard	.3-oz. slice	7
SALISBURY STEAK, frozen		
Morton		
Regular		
Dinner	11-oz. dinner	52
Entree	5-oz. pkg.	35
Country Table	15-oz. dinner	58
King Size		
Dinner	19-oz. dinner	125
Entree	10.3-oz. dinner	87
Stouffer's Lean Cuisine, with		
Italian style sauce & vegetables	9½-oz. pkg.	95
SALMON		
Sockeye, Red or Blueback		
Raw, meat only	4 oz.	40
Canned, solids & liq.	½ cup (4 oz.)	140
Unspecified kind of salmon, baked or broiled with vegetable shortening	4.2 oz. steak (approx. 4″ × 3″ × ½″)	53
SALT, regular or substitute	Any quantity	0
SANDWICH SPREAD		
Hellmann's	1 T. (.5 oz.)	3
Oscar Mayer	1-oz. serving	11
SARDINE, ATLANTIC, canned, in oil		
Solids & liq.	3¾-oz. can	127
Drained solids	3¾-oz. can	129
SAUCE		
Regular		
Barbecue, Open Pit, General Foods	Any quantity	0
Soy, La Choy	1 T. (.5 oz.)	Tr.
Tartar	1 T. (.5 oz.)	7

Food and Description	Measure or Quantity	Cholesterol (milligrams)
Hellmann's	1 T. (.5 oz.)	5
White, home recipe		
Thin	¼ cup (2.2 oz.)	9
Medium	¼ cup (2.5 oz.)	9
Thick	¼ cup (2.2 oz.)	8
Worcestershire, Lea & Perrins	1 T. (.6 oz.)	0
Dietetic		
Barbecue, Estee	1 T. (.6 oz.)	0
Cocktail, Estee	1 T. (.5 oz.)	0
SAUCE MIX, Kikkoman, sweet & sour or teriyaki	Any quantity	0
SAUERKRAUT, canned	Any quantity	0
SAUERKRAUT JUICE, canned, 2% salt	½ cup (4.3 oz.)	0
SAUSAGE		
Pork		
Jimmy Dean	2-oz. serving	48
*Oscar Mayer		
Little Friers	1 link	18
Patty, Southern Brand	1 oz.	18
Smoked, Oscar Mayer		
Beef	1½-oz. link	30
Cheese	1½-oz. link	30
Meat	2-oz. link	68
SAUTERNE, Great Western	3 fl. oz.	0
SCALLION (See **ONION, GREEN**)		
SCALLOP		
Raw, muscle only	4-oz. serving	40
Steamed	4-oz. serving	60
Frozen, Stouffer's Lean Cuisine, oriental, & vegetable with rice	11-oz. pkg.	20
SESAME NUT MIX, canned, Planters, oil-roasted	1 oz.	0

Food and Description	Measure or Quantity	Cholesterol (milligrams)
SESAME SEEDS, dry	Any quantity	0
SHAKE 'N BAKE, General Foods		
Chicken, original, or barbeque	1 envelope	Tr.
Crispy country mild	1 envelope	Tr.
Fish	1 envelope	Tr.
Italian	1 envelope	1
Pork		
Original	1 envelope	0
Barbeque	1 envelope	Tr.
SHALLOT, raw	Any quantity	0
SHERBET, Orange	Any quantity	0
SHREDDED OATS	Any quantity	0
SHREDDED WHEAT	Any quantity	0
SHRIMP		
Raw		
Whole	1 lb. (weighed in shell)	470
Meat only	4 oz.	170
Canned, dry pack, or drained, Bumble Bee, solids & liq.	4 oz.	192
SMOKED SAUSAGE (See **SAUSAGE**)		
SMURF BERRY CRUNCH, cereal, Post	1 cup (1 oz.)	Tr.
SNACK (See **CRACKER, POTATO CHIP,** etc.)		
SNO BALL, Hostess	1½-oz. piece	2
SOFT DRINK, any flavor	6 fl. oz.	0
SOUFFLE, cheese, home recipe	4 oz.	189
SOURSOP, raw	Any quantity	0
SOYBEAN	Any quantity	0
SOYBEAN GRITS, high-fat	1 cup (4.9 oz.)	0
SOYBEAN MILK		
Fluid	4 oz.	0

Food and Description	Measure or Quantity	Cholesterol (milligrams)
Powder	1 oz.	0
SOYBEAN PROTEIN	1 oz.	0
SOYBEAN PROTEINATE	1 oz.	0
SOYBEAN SPROUT (See **BEAN SPROUT**)		
SPAGHETTI		
Cooked		
8–10 minutes, "Al Dente"	1 cup (5.1 oz.)	0
14–20 minutes, tender	1 cup (4.9 oz.)	0
Canned, & meatballs in tomato sauce	1 cup (8.8 oz.)	39
Frozen		
Morton		
Casserole, & meat	8-oz. casserole	25
Dinner, & meatball	11-oz. dinner	27
Stouffer's Lean Cuisine, with beef & mushroom sauce	11½-oz. pkg.	20
SPAGHETTI SAUCE, CANNED		
Regular pack		
Garden Style, Ragú	4-oz. serving	0
Home style, Ragú		
Plain or mushroom	4-oz. serving	0
Meat-flavored	4-oz. serving	2
Marinara, Ragú	4-oz. serving	0
Meat or meat-flavored, Ragú, regular or extra Thick & Zesty	4-oz. serving	2
Meatless or plain		
Hain, Italian style	4-oz. serving	0
Ragú		
Regular	4-oz. serving	0
Extra Thick & Zesty	4-oz. serving	0
Mushroom		
Hain	4-oz. serving	0

Food and Description	Measure or Quantity	Cholesterol (milligrams)
Ragú		
Regular	4-oz. serving	0
Extra Thick & Zesty	4-oz. serving	0
Dietetic pack, Featherweight	⅔ cup	0
SPINACH		
Raw or canned	Any quantity	0
Frozen, Birds Eye		
Chopped or leaf	⅓ of 10-oz. pkg.	0
Creamed	⅓ of 10-oz. pkg.	Tr.
& water chestnuts with selected seasonings	⅓ of 10-oz. pkg.	0
SQUASH SEEDS, dry	Any quantity	0
SQUASH, SUMMER	Any quantity	0
SQUASH, WINTER	Any quantity	0
*START, instant breakfast drink	½ cup	0
STRAWBERRY		
Fresh	Any quantity	0
Frozen, Birds Eye	Any quantity	0
STRAWBERRY JELLY	Any quantity	0
*STUFFING MIX, Stove Top	½ cup	21
SUCCOTASH	Any quantity	0
SUCKER, CARP, raw	Any quantity	0
SUGAR, any type	Any quantity	0
SUGAR SUBSTITUTE		
Estee	1 tsp. (4 grams)	0
Sweet'n It, Dia-Mel, liquid	5 drops	0
SUNFLOWER SEED, raw or roasted	Any quantity	0
SUZY Q, Hostess		
Banana	2¼-oz. piece	22
Chocolate	2¼-oz. piece	16
SWAMP CABBAGE	Any quantity	0
SWEETBREADS, beef		
Raw	1 lb.	1134

Food and Description	Measure or Quantity	Cholesterol (milligrams)
Braised	4 oz.	528
SWEET POTATO, fresh, canned, or frozen	Any quantity	0
SYRUP (See also **TOPPING**)		
Regular		
Cane	Any quantity	0
Corn	1 T. (.7 oz.)	0
Maple	1 T. (.7 oz.)	0
Pancake or waffle		
Log Cabin		
Regular, country kitchen, or maple honey	1 T. (.7 oz.)	0
Buttered	1 T. (.7 oz.)	2
Mrs. Butterworth's	1 T. (.7 oz.)	1

T

Food and Description	Measure or Quantity	Cholesterol (milligrams)
TAMARIND, fresh	Any quantity	0
*TANG	Any quantity	0
TANGELO, fresh	Any quantity	0
TANGERINE or **MANDARIN ORANGE**	Any quantity	0
*TANGERINE JUICE, frozen, Minute Maid	6 fl. oz.	0
TAPIOCA, dry, Minute, quick-cooking	1 T. (.3 oz.)	0
TARO, raw	Any quantity	0
*TEA, bag, canned, instant, or mix	Any quantity	0
*TEXTURED VEGETABLE PROTEIN, Morningstar Farms, any type	Any quantity	0
THURINGER, Oscar Mayer Regular	.8-oz. slice	21

Food and Description	Measure or Quantity	Cholesterol (milligrams)
Beef	.8-oz. slice	17
TIGER TAILS, Hostess	2¼-oz. piece	27
TOMATO, fresh or canned	Any quantity	0
TOMATO JUICE	Any quantity	0
TOMATO PASTE, canned	Any quantity	0
TOMATO PUREE, canned	Any quantity	0
TOPPING, WHIPPED		
Regular		
Cool Whip, Birds Eye		
Dairy	1 T.	Tr.
Nondairy	1 T.	Tr.
Dover Farms, dairy	1 T. (.2 oz.)	<1
Lucky Whip, aerosol	1 T.	0
Whip Topping, Rich's	¼ oz.	0
*Mix		
Regular, Dream Whip	1 T. (.2 oz.)	Tr.
Dietetic		
D-Zerta	1 T.	Tr.
Estee	1 T. (.1 oz.)	0
TOWEL GOURD, raw	Any quantity	0
TROUT, rainbow, fresh, meat & skin	4 oz.	62
TUNA, canned		
In oil		
Solids & liq.	6½-oz. can	100
Drained solids	6½-oz. can	102
In water, solids & liq.	6½-oz. can	116
TUNA PIE, frozen, Morton	8-oz. pie	33
TURKEY		
Raw		
Ready-to-cook	1 lb. (weighed with bones)	272
Dark meat	4 oz.	86

Food and Description	Measure or Quantity	Cholesterol (milligrams)
Light meat	4 oz.	68
Skin only	4 oz.	125
Packaged, Oscar Mayer, breast, sliced	¾-oz. slice	8
Roasted		
Flesh, skin & giblets	From 13½-lb. raw, ready-to-cook turkey	3864
Flesh & skin	From 13½-lb. raw, ready-to-cook turkey	3283
Flesh & skin	4 oz.	105
Meat only		
Light	1 slice (4″ × 2″ × ¼″, 3 oz.)	32
Dark	1 slice (2½″ × 1⅝″ × ¼″, .7 oz.)	21
Skin only	1 oz.	36
TURKEY DINNER OR ENTREE, FROZEN, Morton		
Regular		
Dinner	11-oz. dinner	66
Entree	5-oz. entree	27
Country Table, sliced	15-oz. dinner	45
King Size	19-oz. dinner	75
TURKEY GIZZARD		
Raw	4 oz.	164
Simmered	4 oz.	260
TURKEY PIE, frozen		
	8-oz. pie	20
Morton	8-oz. pie	45
TURNIP	Any quantity	0

Food and Description	Measure or Quantity	Cholesterol (milligrams)
TURNIP GREENS, leaves & stems	Any quantity	0
TWINKIE, Hostess		
Regular	1½-oz. piece	21
Devil's food	1½-oz. piece	10

V

Food and Description	Measure or Quantity	Cholesterol (milligrams)
VEAL, medium fat		
Chuck		
Raw	1 lb. (weighed with bone)	258
Braised, lean & fat	4 oz.	115
Flank		
Raw	1 lb. (weighed with bone)	319
Stewed, lean & fat	4 oz.	115
Foreshank		
Raw	1 lb. (weighed with bone)	168
Stewed, lean & fat	4 oz.	115
Loin		
Raw	1 lb. (weighed with bone)	267

Food and Description	Measure or Quantity	Cholesterol (milligrams)
Broiled, medium done, chop, lean & fat	4 oz.	115
Plate		
Raw	1 lb. (weighed with bone)	264
Stewed, lean & fat	4 oz.	115
Rib		
Raw, lean & fat	1 lb. (weighed with bone)	248
Roasted, medium done, lean & fat	4 oz.	115
Round & rump		
Raw	1 lb. (weighed with bone)	248
Broiled, steak or cutlet, lean & fat	4 oz. (weighed without bone)	115
VEAL DINNER, frozen, Morton, parmigiana		
Regular		
Dinner	11-oz. dinner	36
Entree	5-oz. pkg.	24
Family Meal	2-lb. pkg.	196
King Size	20-oz. dinner	72
VEGETABLES, MIXED		
Canned, regular pack, La Choy, drained, Chinese	⅓ of 14-oz. can	Tr.
Frozen, Birds Eye		
Regular		
Broccoli, cauliflower, & carrots in butter sauce	⅓ of 10-oz. pkg.	6
Broccoli, cauliflower, & carrots in cheese sauce	⅓ of 10-oz. pkg.	3
Broccoli, cauliflower, & red		

Food and Description	Measure or Quantity	Cholesterol (milligrams)
pepper	⅓ of 10-oz. pkg.	0
Carrots, peas, & onions, deluxe	⅓ of 10-oz. pkg.	0
Medley, in butter sauce	⅓ of 10-oz. pkg.	4
Mixed	⅓ of 10-oz. pkg.	9
Mixed, with onion sauce	⅓ of 8-oz. pkg.	Tr.
Peas, & potatoes in cream sauce	⅓ of 8-oz. pkg.	1
Farm Fresh		
Broccoli, carrots, & water chestnuts	⅕ of 16-oz. pkg.	0
Broccoli, cauliflower, & carrot strips	⅕ of 16-oz. pkg.	0
Broccoli, corn, & red pepper	⅕ of 16-oz. pkg.	0
Broccoli, green beans, onions, & red pepper	⅕ of 16-oz. pkg.	0
Brussels sprouts, cauliflower, & carrots	⅕ of 16-oz. pkg.	0
Cauliflower, green beans, & corn	⅕ of 16-oz. pkg.	0
Green beans, corn, carrots, & pearl onions	⅕ of 16-oz. pkg.	0
Green beans, cauliflower, & carrots	⅕ of 16-oz. pkg.	0
Peas, carrots, & pearl onions	⅕ of 16-oz. pkg.	0
International		
Bavarian style beans spaetzle	⅓ of 10-oz. pkg.	12
Chinese style	⅓ of 10-oz. pkg.	Tr.
Far Eastern style	⅓ of 10-oz. pkg.	Tr.
Italian style	⅓ of 10-oz. pkg.	0
Japanese style	⅓ of 10-oz. pkg.	Tr.
Mexican style	⅓ of 10-oz. pkg.	0
New England style	⅓ of 10-oz. pkg.	Tr.

Food and Description	Measure or Quantity	Cholesterol (milligrams)
San Francisco style	⅓ of 10-oz. pkg.	Tr.
Stir Fry		
Chinese style	⅓ of 10-oz. pkg.	0
Japanese style	⅓ of 10-oz. pkg.	0
VERMOUTH	Any quantity	0
VICHY WATER, Schweppes	Any quantity	0
VINEGAR, any type	Any quantity	0

W

Food and Description	Measure or Quantity	Cholesterol (milligrams)
WAFFLE, frozen, Roman Meal		
Regular	1 waffle	4
Golden Delight	1 waffle	13
WAFFLE SYRUP (See **SYRUP**)		
WALNUT	Any quantity	0
WATER CHESTNUT, CHINESE	Any quantity	0
WATERMELON, fresh	Any quantity	0
WAX GOURD, raw	Any quantity	0
WELSH RAREBIT, home recipe	1 cup (8.2 oz.)	72
WESTERN DINNER, frozen, Morton	11.8-oz. dinner	52
WHEAT GERM, crude	Any quantity	0
WHEAT GERM CEREAL	Any quantity	0
WHEAT, ROLLED	Any quantity	0

Y

Food and Description	Measure or Quantity	Cholesterol (milligrams)
YAM	Any quantity	0
YEAST	Any quantity	0
YOGURT		
Regular		
Plain, Dannon	8-oz. container	15
Apple		
Dannon, Dutch	8-oz. container	20
Melangé	6-oz. container	6
Banana, Dannon	8-oz. container	20
Blueberry		
Dannon	8-oz. container	20
Melangé	6-oz. container	6
Cherry		
Dannon	8-oz. container	20
Melangé	6-oz. container	6
Coffee, Dannon	8-oz. container	11
Lemon, Dannon	8-oz. container	11

Food and Description	Measure or Quantity	Cholesterol (milligrams)
Peach, Dannon	8-oz. container	20
Piña colada, Dannon	8-oz. container	20
Pineapple, Melangé	6-oz. container	6
Raspberry		
Dannon, red	8-oz. container	20
Melangé	6-oz. container	6
Strawberry		
Dannon	8-oz. container	20
Melangé	6-oz. container	6
Vanilla, Dannon	8-oz. container	11
Frozen, hard		
Banana, Dannon, Danny-in-a-Cup	8-oz. cup	8
Boysenberry, Dannon, Danny-on-a-Stick, carob-coated	2½-fl.-oz. bar	5
Chocolate, Dannon		
Danny-in-a-Cup	8-fl.-oz. cup	<10
Danny-on-a-Stick		
Uncoated	2½-fl.-oz. bar	5
Chocolate-coated	2½-fl.-oz. bar	5
Piña colada, Dannon, Danny-in-a-Cup	8-oz. cup	<10
Raspberry, red, Dannon		
Danny-in-a-Cup	8-oz. container	<10
Danny-on-a-Stick, chocolate-coated	2½-fl.-oz. bar	5
Strawberry, Dannon		
Danny-in-a-Cup	8 fl. oz. container	<10
Danny-on-a-Stick, chocolate-coated	2½-fl.-oz. bar	5
Vanilla, Dannon		
Danny-in-a-Cup	8 fl. oz.	<10
Danny-on-a-Stick	2½-fl.-oz. bar	5
Frozen, soft, Dannon, Danny-Yo, all flavors	3½-fl.-oz. serving	5

Cholesterol in Your Diet

Adapted from *Eating for a Healthy Heart*, copyright © by the American Heart Association National Center, 7320 Greenville Avenue, Dallas, TX 75231.

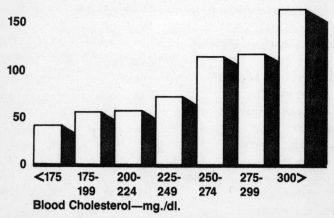

Risk of heart attack increases
AS BLOOD CHOLESTEROL GOES UP
Heart attack rate per 1,000 men per 10 years

Blood Cholesterol—mg./dl.

Fig. 1—Inter-Society Commission for Heart Disease Resources. Atherosclerosis Study Group and Epidemiology Study Group. Primary Prevention of the Atherosclerotic Disease. CIRCULATION, *42.*

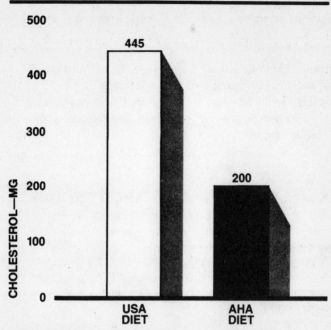

Fig. 2—Comparison of Dietary Cholesterol Intake of Typical U.S. Diet with American Heart Association's Phase 1 Diet Recommendations

SUBSTITUTIONS

Usual Food	Preferred Alternative
High-fat meats	Low-fat meats, fish, and poultry, foods high in vegetable proteins
Egg yolks	Egg whites and egg substitutes
High and medium-fat dairy products	Low-fat and nonfat dairy products

Usual Food	Preferred Alternative
Animal and saturated vegetable fats	Polyunsaturated margarines and oils

Commercial high-fat baked goods and snacks, sugars, sweets and alcohol (reduced when indicated for weight and triglyceride control)	Low-fat, nutritious foods
	  legumes
	  fruits and vegetables
	  breads, cereals, grain products

BREADS, CEREALS AND STARCHY FOODS

Okay Food List

The following is a list of serving sizes to help you in menu planning or calorie control.

Bread, Cereal, Pasta and Starchy Vegetables	Serving Size
Bread—all varieties	1 slice
English muffin, bagel, hamburger bun or large pita bread (each)	½
Tortilla—corn (medium size)	1
Ready-to-eat cereal	⅔ to ¾ cups
Cooked cereal	½ cup
Cooked spaghetti, macaroni, noodles or rice	½ cup
Potato (white), lima beans, green peas or winter squash	½ cup
Corn	⅓ cup
Yam or sweet potato	¼ cup

Crackers and Snacks

Animal crackers	6

Bread sticks (5″ × ½″)	4
Graham crackers (2½″ square)	2
Melba toast (3½″ × 1½″ × ⅛″)	4
Rye crackers	3
Saltines* (2″ square)	6
Oyster crackers*	20
Flatbread or Finn Crisp	4–6
Matzo (6″ square)	1
Pretzels, Dutch,* 3 ring	1
Pretzels,* small 3 ring (1½″ across)	12
Popcorn (popped, no added fat)	1½ cups
Rusks	2
Zwiebach	2

Soup

   1 cup (prepared with water) = 1 serving

Broth or bouillon* (allowed in any amount if sodium is not limited)

Chicken noodle*

Clam chowder, Manhattan-style*

Minestrone*

Onion*

Split pea*

Tomato*

Vegetarian vegetable*

Modified Fat Desserts	Serving Size
2-layer cake, iced	1/12 of cake
Sheet cake, iced	2¼″ × 2½″ × 1½″ piece or 1 serving from 9″ × 13″ pan divided into 20 servings
Cupcake, iced	1 average
Cookies	4 average
Pie, all kinds (double crust)	⅛ of pie

*High in sodium.

1 serving = 1 serving from the Bread, Cereal, Pasta and Starchy Foods group plus 4 teaspoons of fat.

Angel food cake is very low in fat. One-twelfth of a 10-inch tube cake may be substituted for 2 servings from the Bread, Cereal, Pasta and Starchy Foods group.

(Recipes should be modified to contain ingredients from the Okay Food List, such as 1% low-fat or skim milk, margarine, vegetable oil and egg substitute.)

Quick Breads	Serving Size
Banana bread	¹⁄₁₆ of loaf
Biscuits	1 (2″ diameter)
Cornbread	1 muffin or ¹⁄₁₆ of 9″ pan
French toast	1 slice
Muffins	1 average
Pancakes	1 (4″ diameter)
Soft rolls	1 medium roll
Waffles	¼ (1 square) of 9″ waffle

1 serving = 1 serving from the Bread, Cereal, Pasta and Starchy Foods group and 1 teaspoon of fat.

(Recipes should be modified to contain ingredients from the Okay Food List, such as 1% low-fat or skim milk, margarine and egg substitute.)

Foods to Avoid

Items in the following lists should be avoided because of their high-fat and/or high-cholesterol content.

Breads
   Bagels made with eggs or cheese
   Butter rolls
   Cheese breads

Commercial doughnuts, muffins, sweet rolls, biscuits, waffles and
   pancakes
Croissants
Egg breads

Cereals
Granola-type cereals containing coconut or coconut oil

Pastas
Chow mein noodles

Starchy Vegetables
Fried vegetables and those with cream sauce

Crackers
Other commercial crackers such as cheese crackers, butter crackers
and those made with coconut or palm oil

Soup
Cream of potato, mushrooms, chicken, celery, cheese soup
Chunky-type soups
Vichyssoise

Desserts
Cake, commercial
Cheesecake
Pie, commercial
Cookies, commercial
Commercially frozen pie crust
Sweet rolls

Quick Breads
All except those made with allowed ingredients

MILK AND CHEESE

Okay Food List

Milk	Serving Size
Skim or fluid nonfat milk (1% butterfat or less)	1 cup (8 ounces)
Low-fat milk (1% butterfat or less)	1 cup (8 ounces)
Buttermilk made from skim or low-fat milk (1% butterfat or less)	1 cup (8 ounces)
Nonfat or low-fat dry milk (1% butterfat or less)	⅓ cup powder or 1 cup reconstituted
Evaporated skim milk	½ cup undiluted or 1 cup diluted

Creamers
Nondairy creamers made from polyunsaturated fat

Cheese	Serving Size
Dry curd or low-fat cottage cheese	½ cup
Cheeses,* natural or processed, up to 8% butterfat	2 ounces

The nutrition labeling on package should read 2 gm. fat or less per ounce.

Yogurt	Serving Size
Skim or low-fat yogurt, plain	1 cup

---

*High in sodium.

Foods to Avoid

Buttermilk made from whole milk
Cheeses, all varieties made with whole milk or cream
   (containing more than 8% fat)
Chocolate milk
Condensed milk
Cottage cheese, creamed
Cream cheese
Dried whole milk
Evaporated milk
Frozen yogurt made from whole milk
Half and half
Ice cream
Low-fat milk (1½% butterfat or more)
Mellorine
Nondairy coffee creamers (liquid, powdered or frozen)
Nondairy sour creams (tub, powdered or canned)
Nondairy whipped toppings (tub, powdered, aerosol or frozen)
Sour cream
Whipping cream
Whole milk
Yogurt made from whole milk

MEAT, POULTRY AND SEAFOOD

Okay Food List

A maximum of 7 ounces, cooked, per day

- All lean well-trimmed beef, veal, pork and lamb
- All chicken and turkey without skin, including ground turkey

- All fish and shellfish (Since sardines and shrimp are high in cholesterol, a 2-ounce portion is equal to 3 ounces of meat.)
- Wild game—duck, rabbit, pheasant, venison
- Organ meats (Liver, all types—limit to 3 ounces per month since it is very high in cholesterol.)

Foods to Avoid

Beef
All cuts graded Prime or other heavily marbled meats
All untrimmed cuts
Beef sausage
Brisket
Chili meat
Corned beef
Regular ground meat
Pastrami
Plate ribs—short or spare
Rib eye (steak or standing rib roast)

Veal
Breast riblets

Pork, fresh
Boston (roast or steak)
Ground pork
Loin back ribs
Shoulder arm (roast or steak)
Shoulder blade
Sparerib

Pork, smoked (cured)
Bacon
Canned deviled ham
Ham—country, dry cure

Neckbones
Pigs' feet—pickled
Salt pork
Sausage—all kinds
Smoked pork hock
Smoked pork jowl
Smoked pork shoulder, picnic or roll

Lamb
Ground lamb
Mutton

Fish and Shellfish
Caviar
Commercially fried fish or shellfish

Poultry
Poultry skin

Game and Other Meats
Duck, domestic
Goose
Opossum
Raccoon
Venison sausage

Luncheon Meat
Bologna
Canned and packaged luncheon meats
Frankfurters
Headcheese
Salami

Organ Meats
Brains
Chitterlings

Gizzard
Heart
Kidney
Pork maws

Miscellaneous
Commercially fried meat, poultry or seafood
Meats canned or frozen in gravy or sauce
Pork and beans

FATS AND OILS

Okay Food List

Margarines	**Serving Size**
Margarines* listing liquid safflower, corn or sunflower oil as the first ingredient (stick, tub or squeeze)	1 teaspoon
Diet margarine* listing corn, safflower or sunflower oil as the first ingredient	2 teaspoons

Oils	**Serving Size**
Recommended oils, arranged according to highest degree of polyunsaturation	1 teaspoon
Safflower oil	
Sunflower oil	
Corn oil	
Soybean oil	
Cottonseed oil	

*The nutrition labeling should show that there is twice as much polyunsaturated fat as saturated fat in the margarine.

Salad Dressings*	Serving Size
Salad dressing and mayonnaise (commercial or homemade) prepared with allowed oil	2 teaspoons
Low-calorie salad dressings	use as desired

Nuts*	Serving Size
All	1 tablespoon chopped

(1 handful = about ¼ cup or 3 teaspoons fat)

Seeds*	Serving Size
Pumpkin, sesame or sunflower	1 tablespoon

(¼ cup = 4 teaspoons oil)

Avocado	⅛ or 1 tablespoon mashed
Olives*	10 small or 1 tablespoon slices
Peanut Butter*	2 teaspoons

(Can be counted as a fat or meatless alternative.)

Foods to Avoid

All other tub or stick margarine
Margarine listing animal fat (lard or suet)
Bacon drippings
Butter
Chocolate
Coconut, coconut oil, palm or palm kernel oil—usually used in commercial products such as bakery products, nondairy creamers, whipped toppings, candy and commercially fried foods
Gravy made from meat drippings
Ham hocks

---

*High in sodium.

Lard
Meat drippings
Meat fat
Salt pork
Shortening
Suet

Salad Dressing
Blue cheese
Green Goddess
Roquefort
Salad dressings made with sour cream or cheese

Nuts
Cashew
Macadamia
Pistachio

VEGETABLES AND FRUITS

Okay Food List

All vegetables and fruits except those listed below.

Foods to Avoid

Coconut
Avocado
Olives